CIRCLES OF WELLNESS

A GUIDE TO PLANTING, CULTIVATING & HARVESTING WELLNESS

FOR YOU • YOUR FAMILY • YOUR COMMUNITY • YOUR PLANET

Notice: Neither the publisher nor the author is engaged in rendering professional advice or services to the individual reader. The ideas, procedures, and suggestions in this book are not intended as a substitute for consulting a licensed medical professional. All matters regarding your health require medical supervision. Neither the author nor the publisher shall be liable or responsible for any loss or damage allegedly arising from any information or suggestion in this book.

Circles of Wellness: A Guide to Planting, Cultivating & Harvesting Wellness

© 2015 by Queen Afua / Helen O. Robinson

All rights reserved. All rights reserved. No part of this publication may be reproduced, transmitted in any form or by any means, electronic or mechanical, including photocopying, recording, or any other information retrieval system, without the written permission of the publisher, except by a reviewer who may quote brief passages or reproduce illustrations in a review with the appropriate credits.

Cover Design: Metu The Artist
Additional Cover Layout: Cindy Shaw / CreativeDetails.net
Additional Cover Concept: Auset Aswad
Cover Photographer: Keith Major
Hair & Makeup Artist: Daryon Haylock
Master Dance Teacher: Obediah Wright
Text Design, Layout, Graphs & Charts: Cindy Shaw / CreativeDetails.net
Additional Graphs & Charts: Elaine Smith ("Quasheba")
Inside Photography: Auset Aswad, Edfu Katr, Kaiqwon King, Tanco
Inside Artists/Designers:
Global Nation of Wellness Logo, QAWC Catalogue:
Jeff Delerme / Green Studio NYC
Ma'at Scale: Metu The Artist
Product Labels, Queen Afua Wellness Logo, Wellness Warrior Shield Logo:
Rafael Montalvo / www.thinkmontalvo.com
Developmental & Line Editor: Gerianne F. Scott ("Midnight")
Additional Line Editor: Auset Aswad
Co-Editor - Health Care Is Self Care Proposal: Khepera Kearse
Typists: Gerianne Scott, Elaine Smith ("Quasheba")
Tamara Albertini, Tamika Albertini, Sharon Alves
Juanita Myers, Tiffanie S. Perea, Malikah Walters

First Edition
ISBN 978-1512098662

Epigraph

The Way Out Is In

In The Circle Of The Self

In The Circle Of Our Family

In The Circle Of Our Friends

And Our Community

We Don't Give Up, We Go Within
To Our Wellness

Planting Into Our Circles Freedom,
Cultivating What We Want to Receive

Harvesting Health, Joy Happiness,
Peace and Abundance

Reaching The Highest
Of Shai (Karma)

Contents

Dedication ix
Preface xi
Foreword xiii
Acknowledgements xv
Circles of Wellness Daily Affirmation xvii
Global Round Table Gathering (Introduction) xix

Paradigm Shift 1: TRANSFORMATION – Planting Circles for Restoration and Rejuvenation

    The Ultimate Circle I Am 3
    360°: The Process 8
    Circle of Awareness 11
    Holistic Lovemaking 13
    Circle of Intimacy 15
    From Forgiveness to Freedom 18
        Forgiveness Affirmation 20
On the Wings of Forgiveness 21
    Get Out of the Box 23
    Circles Reflect Circles 26
    Heal Your Life. Form Circles. 27
    Rejuvenate Our Communities 29
        Plant * Cultivate * Agenda * Meditation
    Make It A Million (Chart) 38
    The People Have the Power 39
    Womb Wellness Circles 41
        Awakening Affirmation 43
    Men, Form Your Circles 44
        Man Heal Affirmation 48
    Save Our Children 49
    Addressing Autism 57
    Love Your Children 60
    Uplift Our Elders 61

PARADIGM SHIFT 2: UNIFICATON – CULTIVATING ALLOPATHIC AND HOLISTIC CIRCLES

A New Way of Life 70
    It Begins with Doctor Davidson 71
    Both of Them 72
    We Meet 74
    Health Report Card 76
    The CO$T of Not Knowing 78
    Is it Possible? 79
    Health Care Is Self-Care (Excerpts) 81
        Crisis * Statistics * Proposal * *Magnificent Ones*
        Test Case * *Testimonials* * Report
It's Time for a Change 105

PARADIGM SHIFT 3: RESTORATION – CULTIVATING AN EMERALD GREEN LIFESTYLE

    Shift to Green 109
    How Do I Rejuvenate Myself? 111
    The 4 Ps of Optimal Wellness 113
    9 Steps to Holistic Living 114
    84 Day Whole Living Program 116
    Let's Do the Math 118
    Dietary Lifestyles & Meal Plans 120
        Energized Flexitarian * Super Vegetarian
        Raw Vegan * Purified Juiceatarian
    Brain Food 129
    Prepare for Your Journey 131
    Say It Is So (Affirmations) 133
    Write On (Journal) 135
    Check Up (Checklist) 138

PARADIGM SHIFT 4: EMPOWERMENT – USING WELLNESS TOOLS

    Elements, Wheels & Products 143
    Wellness Challenges (Checklist) 145

Product Usage Chart 147
12 Empowerment Wheel Circles 151
Food as Medicine 176
Benefits of Green Life 178
Green Clay – 21 Ways 180
Breathe, Again 183
Your Anatomy, Your Kit 184
12 Points / 21 Days 185

Paradigm Shift 5: REJUVENATION – Harvesting Wellness at Home

Baba Ishangi's Round House Home 188
Set Up Your Home 189
Room Conversions 191
Nutrition Kitchen Pharmacy 192
My Kitchen Is Free From Negativity 193
An Invitation 196
Whole Food Affirmation 197
A Mother's Testimonial 198
Hydrotherapy Bathroom 200
Family Live-In Room 203
Sun Ra Yoga 206
Regeneration Bedroom 210
Now That You Know 212

Next Steps

24 Hour Global Fast 214
Circle of Healers 215
Hip-Hop Medicine Man 217
Crop Circles 219
From Circles to Spirals 220
In the Spirit of Transformation 222

CATALOGUE 223

ONGOING 236

Dedication

I dedicate **Circles of Wellness**
to all those inspired to plant a wellness lifestyle;
to all those seeking to cultivate a life of wholeness;
and to all those who know in their hearts that
they have the ability to harvest a new people; a new planet.

I dedicate **Circles of Wellness**
to the Wellness of our Future Generations;
to our children's children.

Guidance and protection to my granddaughters:
my eldest Atnnt Torain,
and my youngest Maatia Torain.

Preface

$\mathcal{M}$any moons ago I visited Ananda Ashram[1] a Yoga and meditation retreat center in the Catskills Mountains, in upstate New York. I was ending a marriage. Accompanied by my three babies 2, 4 and 6 years old, I was facing a new life. While at the Ashram I heard a song that touched my heart. For more than a quarter of a century, my children and I have hummed the melody. The lyrics stayed with me: *"Circle round the planet… Circle round for peace…"* At the time, I had not collected the names of the title or the writer of the song. Nonetheless, those words have inspired my journey into my power circle. *"Circle round the planet…for our future generations…"* Those words have motivated me to continuously plant and cultivate Circles of Wellness for our future generations.

As I was going over the final edits on this book with my editor, Gerianne , (our Literary "Midnight" Midwife), and Quasheba, an assistant and a new Sacred Woman, I shared with them that a song I heard long ago was a powerful and long-time motivation of my "circle of wellness" philosophy. The two women quickly researched on the Internet and in minutes they told me that actually there were two songs, "Circle Round for Freedom" and "Circle Chant", written by Linda Hirschhorn[2]. Then, they played the songs for me. My eyes were filled with tears; once again, my heart was touched. Clearly, planting, and cultivating, and harvesting circles is my honor and privilege; my life; my Circle of Self.

Circles of Wellness: A Guide to Planting, Cultivating & Harvesting Wellness is a guide to gaining vibrant, healthy living for you, your family, your community and your planet. It raises the questions and offers solutions. This book is divided into five chapters called Paradigm Shifts. Paradigms are what we call "normal" about the way we think and the way we act. Five is the number for balance, freedom and grace. The text is presented in five chapters that teach how to make balanced, graceful paradigm shifts to the freedom of healthy living. It is time to plant new seeds as we rethink and redo our personal and planetary health care. It is time to transform our idea of "normal" away from being stuck in sickness into a new vision of optimal living.

Circles of Wellness: A Guide to Planting, Cultivating & Harvesting Wellness presents the opportunity to become aware of and heal the Circle of Self in order to cultivate and grow circles of wellness in families and communities around the globe. One by one as we activate the strategies of wellness and we choose to live lives based on a natural, holistic, Emerald Green Lifestyle, our paradigms will shift. By shifting to "wellness thinking" and "wellness acting", you, your family, your community and your planet can begin harvesting collective greatness; 360°; full circle!

---

[1] Ananda Ashram in Monroe, New York, is a Yoga retreat and spiritual-educational center founded in 1964 by Shri Brahmananda Sarasvati (then Ramamurti S. Mishra, M.D.) as the country center of the Yoga Society of New York, Inc.

[2] © 1984 Linda Hirschhorn, Kehila Publications (BMI). Music and text of "Circle Round for Freedom" refrain from "Circle Chant" by Linda Hirschhorn. Copyright © 1982, from Gather Round Songbook (Tara Publications), 1988 and the recording Roots and Wings (Oyster Albums, P.O. Box 3929, Berkeley, CA 94703), 1992.

Foreword

I am pleased and proud to endorse this latest edition to the Queen Afua Wellness Library. As a guide Circles of Wellness: A Guide to Planting, Cultivating & Harvesting Wellness is an invaluable tool for the partnership between holistic and traditional care. The more you incorporate its principles, the more the results may be quantified in the world of traditional medicine. In my opinion, its intent is collaborative – and could well be the missing link in the approach to chronic illness. I resubmit Thoughts from the Examination Room I had a few years ago.

Dr. Bernadette L. Sheridan MD F.A.A.F.P

Thoughts from the Examination Room

From the sacred space of the Doctor's Exam Room, where men and women surrender pretense and ego to the desire to find answers, avoid pain and prolong life, I join my voice with my fellow collaborators to repeat the timeliness of this work and the urgency of the situation. I have been a practicing, traditionally trained licensed and Board Certified Family Practitioner for over thirty years. The observations that I have made during that time are, no doubt, reflected around the country – in all communities– rural, urban, upper class, and inner city. As a nation, we are becoming technologically advanced, but these impressive strides are not reflecting in a healthier population. In the 21st Century, people still succumb to the same chronic illness as three decades ago, and at much higher rates. Lack of access to care and information are minor reasons for the quantum leap to near epidemic numbers of Hypertension, Type 2 Diabetes, Heart Disease and Cancer. People fill the clinics and offices in record numbers. At the same time the Internet has made us all "research experts" and prescription drug sales account for billions of dollars in the Health Care Budget. Nonetheless the statistics do not redeem us as a healthier population. The last, chilling piece of the equation, the one that frosts the cake of urgency, is the fact that the children are now joining the ranks of the chronically ill, succumbing to "adult diseases" before they are even old enough to vote. We literally are dying to be well.

The solution, of course, is not found in a single place, but in a collaborative effort of things simple and things complex. There is no turning away from the fact that a lifestyle based on consuming toxic food while growing up; and growing old in a stressful century will require more and more pharmaceutical intervention to suppress its toxic effects. In her previous books Queen Afua offers steps to self-healing, clear thinking, forgiveness and release. The message here continues to be, based on the simple realization that: the car runs better and breaks down less if you fill it with quality fuel and care for it responsibly. Several of her previous templates for healing repeated herein could not be timelier. To self-heal, think clearly, forgive and release together in circles is perhaps the most timely aspect of Queen's message.

Kudos, thanks and professional respect to Queen Afua, whom I have the privilege to know as colleague and friend. From our first encounter, we recognized each other as healers on a common road. Because of that recognition and mutual respect, we have created our "circle" for a common good, proving that, yes, it is possible for holistic strategies and mainstream medical to align. It is my hope and desire that her book provokes most of us to form circles in order to heal together. To transform one by one will ultimately have an effect on all.

Respectfully resubmitted
Bernadette L. Sheridan MD, F.A.A.F.P
(CEO/Founder) Grace Family Medical Practice/Brooklyn, NY

Acknowledgements

I **give thanks for** my ancestors who continue to inspire my life's work as a healer: my father Ephriam Robinson, my grandfather Big Daddy Ford, my grandmother Big Mama Ford and my Master Herbal Teacher, Dr. John E. Moore who taught me first-hand how to "talk to the elements."

For years of Support leading up to this Circle of Work, "Thank you" to my now adult children Supa Nova Slom, Sherease Ma'at, and Ali Amechi. Bob and Muntu Law, "Imhotep" Gary Byrd, Sen-Ur Ankh Ra Semahj Se Ptah, Dr. Jesse Brown, Ellis Liddell, Mother Etta Dixon, Diana Pharr, Lady Prema, Queen Esther Sarr & her husband Baba Sarr, Phyllis Yvonne Stickney Ma'at, Pastor Johnny Ray Youngblood, Sheila Everette Hale, Danyelle Claxton, Kimberly Boyd, Betty Lane, Evangeline Mayweather, Brother Wanique Shabazz, Lloyd Strayhorn, Mut Ast, Empress Tandi, Nati of Afrikan World Books, Nabi Faison, and Mudman of Philly. To all those who challenged me to the core of my being, I am deeply thankful that you have inspired me to go within to my center circle and to find that the power to heal is within me to heal myself and all my relations.

I give thanks to a beautiful and powerful staff: Osayande Angaza, Edfu Katr, Chris "Kazi" Rolle, Sacred Woman Auset, Queen Neith, Totep Knshu, Esther Wade and Debra Ma'at for your support in growing and maintaining the Queen Afua Wellness healing vision for personal, family, community and global wellness; all the Sacred Woman and the Man Heal Thyself Elder Guides; all The Global Nation of Wellness volunteers; the Wellness Warriors ,Womb Wellness Workers and Emerald Green Holistic Practitioners; dedicated volunteers and students; and all who I've met in the world on my journey who have been supportive in any and all ways. Elder Master Teacher Tahar Qaamun Ra Ankh Ka Ptah Alem, **Thank you** for your loving, "hands-on" restoration of the people to wholeness.

I am grateful for Dr. Bernadette Sheridan of Brooklyn, New York and Dr. William Emikola Richardson of Atlanta, Georgia for actively supporting me.

(CIRCLES OF WELLNESS)

Throughout the years, you have been my Circle of Conscious Physicians; for the collective I call "The Healers Circle", who have journeyed with me (and those who will) for the 24 Hour Global Fast Teleconferences. I wish continued strength and blessings for all these wellness advocates.

I am grateful that Oprah Winfrey and Deepak Chopra hosted a 21 Day Meditation; my sister, Iyanla Vazant, took the healing to the streets on OWN TV to help to end sexual oppression and the pathology of racial oppression; Linda Hirschhorn wrote "Circle Round for Freedom", a song which has touched my heart for many years.

For bringing forth this work I am absolutely thankful to my City of Wellness team for your support; Ali Amechi "The Great", The Mayor of the City of Wellness and Founder of the Global Nation of Wellness for his vision and his dedication to its building and growth; "Quasheba" (Elaine Smith) who, as a Sacred Woman, rose to the challenge of assembling this work; Rupert Knight "The Black Knight" for being Founder of Powerful Pioneers, Perry Coleman for hard work and dedication, Jeff Delerme of Green Studio NYC for his loving, creative skills; Auset Aswad for her steadfast genius and dedication to the work; Dee Dee McCalla for deliciously "adding to the soup" with her heart, mind and eyes on the work; Cindy Shaw for her generosity and her dedication to detail and design; Gerianne Scott, the "Literary Midnight Midwife" who, once again, stayed with the "baby" from conception to birth.

I am so thankful for the Circle of Ida Robinson, my mother, who lived to see these times of my work.

...And so it is....
Queen Afua

Circle of Wellness Affirmation

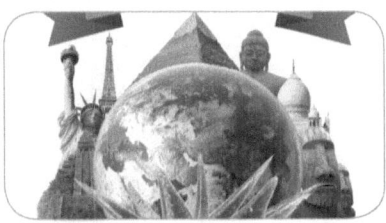

I am a circle of health, joy and happiness, as I eliminate physical,
mental emotional and relationship dis-ease.

I embrace daily, body, mind and spiritual well-being,
as I go within my inner circle to seek relief.

I feed my inner circle with high frequency nourishment,
that is contained in whole foods, healing prayers
and harmonizing meditation and daily self-nurturing acts.

My circle supplies my wellness needs.
When I meet others on the path of wellness,
our circles of wellness are brilliantly magnified.

I am a Circle, radiating optimal wellness steadily growing in health and vitality.

I reach out from deep inside myself to unite with my In-dwelling Healer,
to help create more Circles of Wellness, to overcome global disharmony together.
We are charged and able on life's journey to help uplift family,
friends, and community.

Together we plant, cultivate and harvest the City of Wellness.
We the People make up the city for as we heal the people,
we heal the city in ever-evolving Circles of Wellness.

Queen Afua

Introduction

"Queen Afua's books are "channelings." They are as simple as they are profound. They are divinely inspired directions on how humanity may reclaim health of mind, body and spirit. As always, Queen Afua remains open to receiving guidance from spirit. Through Circles of Wellness, once again she reveals what is revealed (channeled) to her regarding a guide for us to get back to our origins of well being on a global scale. In circular mode, from her circle of self, Queen Afua shares and connects with all other circles of self (you and me and all). Geometrically (and alchemically) speaking these connections interlock and vibrate on to spherical dimensions."

DIANA PHARR/SPIRITUAL TEACHER
(& LONG-TIME SISTER-FRIEND)

Gather At The Global Round Table

We are gathered at a round table because it is a circle and everything we need is here. Throughout our global history we have gathered in circles to share family events, conduct rituals and celebrate cultural rites. In circles, facing the ocean, at riversides, in forests and on mountaintops, humans have assembled to express our minds and soothe our souls. Circles have been familiar meeting arrangements on all continents, because the ancestors in our indigenous populations understood the power of convening in circles to share ideas and demonstrate unity. Whether we call them jamborees, pow-wows, prayer circles, drum circles or study groups, none of us are new to circle assembly. We are gathered at this Global Round Table because everything we need is here, in this circle.

CIRCLES OF WELLNESS

Immediately, we need solutions to our trans-global concerns regarding life-sustaining resources and our mutual access to them. We need to address everyone's right to breathe clean air, drink and bathe in clean water, grow and eat uncompromised plants and to coexist with the other living creatures in our respective environments. The questions raised and the solutions acted upon will have both immediate and lasting impacts, not only on us, but more importantly on the future generations we hope will survive our decisions. Politically, socially, economically, physically, mentally and metaphysically, our decisions and actions have consequences. What we say and do from this moment of our individual and collective consciousness is critical to what happens next… in every circle of our lives.

We have been warned. According to citations in the Ancient Mayan almanac and prophecies made by many global philosophers it has been predicted that humanity will experience a planetary shift of great magnitude. We have seen these predictions come to be. On our planet the increase of earthquakes, floods and hurricanes challenge the quality of life and destroy large populations of humanity at an alarming rate. In urban, rural and remote settings we are concerned about the economy, the safety and education of our children, our ability to protect and support our families and our opportunity to co-exist peacefully with our neighbors. We need to talk about how our urban youth are regularly being incarcerated as the norm; and about the violence occurring in the home; and the violence occurring in the streets. We need to talk about health and health care. Globally, people are stressed, oppressed, and depressed. Although technology is expanding, people are still getting sicker – filled with mental, physical, and emotional dis-ease. Hospitals are closing. Where health insurance is available, the cost is rising. Certainly, it is the right time for us and our families to gather at a Global Round Table to voice our needs about our physical, mental, emotional and spiritual wellness.

Over the past four decades I have written books in which are provided "greenprints" for living an Emerald Green Lifestyle. In all the books are holistic tools and strategies for using food, herbs, the elements, meditations,

(INTRODUCTION)

affirmations, teachings from ancient Nile Valley wisdom and methods of detoxification and purification to facilitate restoration of the body, mind and spirit. I bring these to the Global Round Table. In **Heal Thyself for Health and Longevity,** are the initial steps and recipes for establishing a holistic lifestyle. My motivation for writing **Sacred Woman: A Guide to Healing the Feminine Body, Mind, and Spirit** was to reach out to women, and to encourage each one to know herself and to love herself. The strategies focus on creating healing energy especially for use in our relationships. Included are techniques for cultivating sacred words, foods and spaces for our living and working. Next, I wrote, **The City of Wellness: Restoring Your Health Through the Seven Kitchens of Consciousness** which initiated the City of Wellness campaign reminding us that we do not have to live with pain, dis-ease and fear. As individuals healed the entire planet could heal. In **The City of Wellness** individuals could learn to observe the relationship between their food lifestyle and their wellness. All are encouraged to accept accountability for their well-being and invited to participate in the building of the City of Wellness.

Overcoming an Angry Vagina: Journey to Womb Wellness is a self-help guide for empowerment especially regarding womb issues. the majority of us, here at the Global Round Table realize that, "If Mama ain't happy *(well},* nobody is happy *(well).*" We recognize that if there is pain and dis-ease in a woman's womb, her physical seat of reproduction, and in the womb of her heart and her mind and her spirit; if she is not well, her relationships, also, will not be well. Her womb damage affects interactions with her mate and her children and her work and her attempts to seek joy. That global wellness is completely connected to womb wellness is being accepted as, "…and so it is." In Divine Order, the men asked for guidance specifically written for them. My sons, Ali Ameche Torain and Supa Nova Slom, each a Wellness Warrior and Healing Juggernaut for over two decades, convinced me that I had to write, **Man Heal Thyself** which provides the men with the techniques unique to their wellness quest. And so we arrive at this time and in this place. The need is for intensive application of all we have been learning, as we continue be in the circles of our lives. It is time for high frequency activation of "wellness work" in order to heal our planet.

(CIRCLES OF WELLNESS)

We are gathered at this Global Round Table because everything we need is here. We are seriously in need of a paradigm shift, (a change, a transformation) of how we look at and obtain body, mind and spiritual detoxification and rejuvenation. We must shift from accepting dis-ease to preparing for wellness in all aspects of our lives. We must STOP; TAKE DEEP CLEANSING BREATHS and ASK: *WHAT CAN I DO?* The prophecies of old advised that those who are spiritually, mentally and physically toxic will suffer greatly; and those who purify and are holistically prepared will be lifted to great heights. *Are we prepared?* At this critical threshold, I suggest that we must make paradigm shifts in our approach to wellness. It is time to rethink and redo our personal and planetary health care. It is time to transform our idea of "normal" away from being stuck in sickness into a new vision of wellness. I bring to the Global Round Table, **Circles of Wellness: A Guide to Planting, Cultivating & Harvesting Wellness,** presented in five chapters called Paradigm Shifts to suggest how to make balanced, graceful transitions to the freedom of healthy living. (Five is the number for balance, freedom and grace.)

Paradigm Shift 1: TRANSFORMATION – Planting Circles for Restoration and Rejuvenation begins with acknowledging the Circle of Self and the circles in our lives. It introduces The Process of determining whether a particular circle we are in is one of confusion or one of balance. The Process includes Wellness Work to guide us to awareness and then forgiveness. We must forgive all who have caused us pain and hurt, including ourselves. Forgiving is no simple transformation, especially if undertaken alone. Therefore, I suggest planting seeds of wellness by forming circles of wellness to heal ourselves and our families and our communities. Planting circles of wellness is the process of wrapping healing hands and hearts around each of us on the planet. Planting circles of wellness is the logical and loving beginning of the mission to harvest personal, family, community, and global healing.

Paradigm Shift 2: UNIFICATION – Cultivating Allopathic and Holistic Circles contains the story of Dr. Bernadette Sheridan (allopathic approach) and I, Queen Afua (holistic approach) coming together to examine our techniques for achieving wellness. In a history-making clinical study we asked and answered the question: *Is it possible for us to work side by side to increase wellness in our community?* Within the chapter are excerpts of the proposal and the report of my program: "Health Care Is Self Care." It was tested on participants called the Magnificent **Ones** for an 84 Day study holistically conducted by me and clinically supported by Dr. Sheridan. **Paradigm Shift 3: RESTORATION – Cultivating an Emerald Green Lifestyle** revisits my ongoing strategies for detoxification and purification to heal thyself, our families, our communities and ultimately, our planet. Each strategy supports the paradigm for a planetary shift to restoration.

Paradigm Shift 4: EMPOWERMENT – Using Wellness Tools, includes a wellness self-assessment worksheet and strategies and techniques for using the elements to support cultivation on the journey to wellness. Additionally, there are guides and illustrations of the 12 Empowerment Wheel Circles (formerly Wellness Empowerment Wheels). There are empowerment wheels for the Breast, Prostate, Blood and Bones, Emotions, Skin and more. These address wellness challenges including: Diabetes, High Blood Pressure, Fibroid Tumors and Obesity.

Paradigm Shift 5: REJUVENATION – Harvesting Wellness at Home is a guide to creating a wellness home based on Baba Kwame Ishangi's Wellness Round House Home in Sene-Gambia, West Africa. There are suggestions for converting your home into a rejuvenation center and incorporating appropriate affirmations, guides and charts to support your paradigm into optimal wellness preparation and usage of your home. Lovingly submitted are the instructions for creating your Nutrition Kitchen Pharmacy, your Hydrotherapy Bathroom, your Family Live-In Room (for Meditation, Study, Exercise, and Yoga) and your Regeneration Bedroom. By shifting to thinking and acting in wellness, you, your family, your community, and your planet can begin harvesting collective greatness, 360 degrees, full circle!

Finally, in a post script section of **Circles of Wellness is Next Steps.** This section introduces a few participants from the Circle of Healers and their work, especially as presented on the free 24 Hour Global Fast Teleconference. The 24 Hour

(CIRCLES OF WELLNESS)

Global Fast was created to celebrate each equinox and solstice. Under the title: *The Day That Healed the World* a Circle of Healers gathers on the call to answer the question: *What would you do to heal planet Earth?* Nearly 100 healers have presented responses offering their ideas for healing ourselves and the earth. From Naturopaths and Musicians to Wealth Advisors and Medical Doctors, healers in all fields provide thought-provoking and healing comments. (See the link in the back of the book for further contact to this amazing Circle of Healers and connect to ongoing and healing conversation.)

 We are gathered at this Global Round Table because everyone who needs to be is here in the circle. We are those who feel helpless, hopeless….powerless; and those who have made the paradigm shift to embrace the empowerment to Heal Thyself. We are gathered knowing each of us has something to bring and something to do. We are here with our obesity and with our famine. While some of us here are victims of inequalities based on race, religion, ethnicity, gender and gender-preference choices; some of us here are beneficiaries of racial, gender, class and/or wealth privilege. Because we have in common global citizenship, we have in common global responsibility to overcome dis-harmony and raise our frequency to peace. All of us, including those of us called "Baby Boomers", must choose now to, "Purify or die." Collectively, we must choose to live lives based on, "Health Care Is Self Care". The philosophy of **Circles of Wellness** involves the connectivity of all of our acts of oneness unified for the common good. Imagine everyone around you experiencing an exuberant lifestyle of wellness! Imagine harvesting disease-free homes and neighborhoods, towns, cites and nations completely liberated from illness. I clearly see that vision as a new world of wellness.

We must honestly search within ourselves for the challenges that "trap" us in boxes of non-growth and dis-ease. We must forgive ourselves and each other for whatever pain and hurt we caused. We must actively make paradigm shifts by looking at things differently and doing things differently. WE HAVE THE POWER to transform the fate of the planet and all who share existence on it. If you are reading these pages it is not necessary for you or yours to be sick; nor to live in a

(INTRODUCTION)

home that does not support your well-being in every way. We can actively make vibrant, healthy decisions to form circles that share the light of a natural-living lifestyle. We, the People can make powerful changes by shifting our paradigm from accepting illness to expecting and creating wellness. We must aim for there to be global millions able to choose to live healthy lives; from the microcosm to the macrocosm, we each have the ability to plant and cultivate the seeds In order to grow Circles of Wellness.

It begins with YOU! You must make the journey onto the path of purification through the seasonal One Day Fasting Detox Program and continue your wellness quest onto the path of the Emerald Green 21 Day Detox Program (presented in Paradigm Shift 3). Embrace this text as your passport to The Global Circle of Wellness. Use it as the guide to make the paradigm shift away from dis-ease, forward to our global decrease of the epidemics of cancer, diabetes, asthma, high blood pressure, fibroid tumors, obesity, depression, and AIDS. We are on our way to global wellness with the 12 Empowerment Wheel Circles and with high frequency nourishment and liberation consciousness from nutrition kitchens where food is our medicine and life is worth living. Our immune systems will improve when our bodies are purified from toxicity. When we STOP EATING DEATH, such as, flesh, micro-waved, chemically-injected, denatured, seedless, GMO and "fast" foods and instead, those who are able to choose, *do* choose to eat, LIVE, whole, organic foods, we will restore our bodies, minds and hearts. From your Circles of Wellness, by your example, you can invite your families and friends. As they accept, more new circles of wellness will be created. Just like trillions of cells make up the body's anatomy, hundreds, upon thousands, upon millions of people will unite to make up the Global Nation of Wellness. As the people cleanse, one by two by twenty families and communities and circles will detoxify. Disease is spread by toxic thoughts and toxic lifestyles. Wellness can be spread by holistic thoughts and holistic lifestyles within the body, within the communities, throughout the world.

When we are in harmony with nature, we are in harmony with ourselves. Healthy people can look forward to creating healthy relationships. In Circles of Wellness, we can begin to end violence in the home and violence in the world. People in Circles of Wellness, can formulate creative solutions for transforming our global wellness one person, one circle and one community at a time. Fellow Humans, we are gathered here, at the Global Round Table facing worldwide challenges and facing each other. It is our time to be victorious in our journey and to harvest Global Wellness and Global Harmony.

THE POWER TO HEAL IS WITHIN US!

(PARADIGM SHIFT 1)

TRANSFORMATION

Planting Circles for Restoration and Rejuvenation

"Transformation to higher ground –
Transformation to a higher place."

Katriel Wise, Metaphysical Music Medicine Man

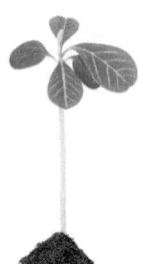

(TRANSFORMATION)

THE ULTIMATE CIRCLE I AM

There are 360 degrees in a complete circle. I have found that there are complete circles of confusion and there are complete circles of balance and like most people, I live between these two types of circles of life. During forty years of holistic living and practitioner work I have opened and closed ten wellness centers in my community. I have survived fires, floods and having a padlock placed by the sheriff on my business and my home. At the same times these challenges were occurring, I gave birth three times; each time by way of Caesarean section. As each birth almost took my life, each one also made me more convicted to heal myself. I have been married three times. Each marriage led me to the brink of enlightenment and deeper into my inner soul self-circle of reflection. Throughout the years I began and ended new circles with friends, family and strangers.

Your circle tells your story, your journey. Circles are not static; they move and expand, spiraling up and down depending on one's consciousness. Circles are mystical, evolving and growing as one evolves and grows. One may think about circles as finite and say "I am finally here, I have arrived. I am complete", until… the next evolution! Circles can act as rain that cleanses; a monsoon or a blizzard that destroys; or, if we allow it, as an ocean wave that propels one toward growth. When the circles act as an ocean wave it moves us forward. No matter what circle you find yourself in, always dwell there with a "light heart." It will lead you to discover that the ultimate circle is you. Circles talk, strengthen; give and take. Circles reflect your aspirations, your hopes and dreams. Your circle may seem to be falling apart before your eyes and everyone in your circle may seem to be against you. Doors close; dams and bridges are destroyed and it seems there is no way out. Now, when you are in the eye of the hurricane… stop, listen and run to your Center Circle for refuge. Your Center Circle resides within! Your Center Circle is that deep, quite, watchful, peace-filled inner space;

the wisdom core of your true essence. Receive the message your authentic self speaks to you as it transforms your inner and outer world into the light of truth, justice and harmony.

One of my most challenging circles, which, therefore, brought a most important lesson, occurred within my family circle. For many years a family member adamantly scorned my holistic philosophy and ridiculed my wellness work. This person threatened to figure out a way to close down my wellness center. Nonetheless, from within my circle of cultivating wellness, every day I got up and continued my work. Clients continued to seek consultations from me. I continued to develop wellness formulas, study holistic techniques from master practitioners, improve strategies and train Wellness Warriors to become qualified consultants and practitioners. In 2009, the then Brooklyn Borough President Marty Markowitz honored me with a Proclamation declaring June 27 Annual Queen Afua Day in Brooklyn, New York City. My Circle of Wellness Care was thriving. Meanwhile, the family member who threatened to destroy my work recently called and asked for my help with challenging health issues. A wise and trusted friend advised me to direct my family member to become a client *but only* under the care of a practitioner other than myself. A month later, under the professional guidance of one of the Wellness Warriors and after taking the suggested formulas the former opponent called to tell me they were feeling better and getting better. Clearly, this person's Circle of Self was evolving to a "heal thyself" state of body and mind. This is just one example of two circles – one of confusion; one of balance– growing, shifting, colliding, and changing in a life; my life. Circles are constant in one's life; they have certainly been constant in mine. It is clear to me that I live between the two types of circles; we all do.

The circle is **Sacred Geometry.** Based on Nile Valley teachings the symbol for the circle is the sun disc or sunlight. Sunlight gives energy, enlightens, nourishes, nurtures and heals. If you open up to the lessons that the circle brings you will receive the wisdom of the circle. According to the ancient Nile Valley teachings your Center Circle is the place called MA'AT. It is the place where great ones go to protect, refuel, and realign their body, mind and spirit with illuminating

(Transformation)

possibilities. Nelson Mandela resided within his Center Circle and continued to fight for the freedom of the people even though he was imprisoned behind bars by South African apartheid. Mahatma Gandhi lived within his Center Circle while he fought for social justice. Sojourner Truth, Martin Luther King, Malcolm X, Fannie Lou Hammer, and most certainly, Sister Harriet Tubman, each dwelled within their Center Circle as each dedicated their life to the cause of freedom and justice. From that unshakeable, unbreakable place of inner refuge they tapped into their natural greatness and gave hope to the people who looked for the Promised Land. No matter what challenges you meet in your circles, breathe deeply, listen and relax completely as you allow yourself to be guided into your all knowingness and right direction, from circle to circle.

From the time of conception within our mother's wombs and throughout our lives we are in circles. Your circle is you. Each of the circles you enter gives you an opportunity to heal, to advance yourself to higher ground; to overcome. As a child in my parents' home, I was comforted within my mother's circle. My Mother's Circle primarily existed in the kitchen. The kitchen was the center circle where homework was done while my mom spoke to friends on the phone as she braided my hair. In the kitchen T.V. was watched, while all meals were prepared and served. Throughout my youth I was in a dietary circle of dis-ease, discomfort and discontent as I feasted on the "All American toxic lifestyle." (See: *The City of Wellness: Restoring Your Health Through the Seven Kitchens of Consciousness* by Queen Afua.) In my mother's kitchen the family enjoyed macaroni and cheese, candied yams, collard greens – with fat back and fried chicken throughout the week. Every Friday before sun down dinner was fried fish with canned peas and corn bread. Mama's good home-cooking gave me her love from and in her kitchen. For sixteen years I lived in a circle of dietary manslaughter in the form of everything from peanut butter and jelly on white bread, to pork chops and steak dinners, topped off with mashed potatoes and butter, chased down by Kool-Aid (tap water, sugar and red dye #2). My family circle was well fed toxicity and thus I became plagued with asthma, allergies, PMS, headaches, mood swings, eczema and stress. Although there was always plenty to eat, I was malnourished and my life was closing down on me fast.

(CIRCLES OF WELLNESS)

When I turned 16 in 1969 the explosion of a new circle moving throughout the United States made a huge impact on the world stage. That circle pulled me right out of my circle of ignorance and unconscious toxic thinking, eating and being. It brought me out of my "comfort zone of disease" to all kinds of liberation circles. The people rose up from social unrest and injustice fighting for their freedom. Sweet Honey In the Rock sang, *"We who believe in freedom cannot rest."* Richie Havens (a fellow Brooklynite) opened up at the Woodstock Peace Concert and created the iconic song *"Freedom"* while a million youth listened expecting to find answers to their lives. Pharoah Sanders sang, *"The Creator has a master plan"* and the Freedom Riders from the south rode throughout Ku Klux Klan land, fighting for freedom while being threatened, sprayed, jailed and even murdered. Justice and Equality. The Black Panthers and African Nationalist movements grew throughout the urban cities holding together an unbroken circle of hope *"By any means necessary."* Circles of students from campuses across the country fought to end the war with sit-ins and rallies shouting *"All power to the people."* Many people committed to justice and equality were ready to die for freedom.

In 1969, I woke up and entered into all kinds of circles which liberated me from dis-ease. Holistic health, vegetarian lifestyle and yoga were unleashed in America and I healed myself with their healing fire. In 1969, I began to heal myself culturally as African dancing and drumming swept through the world. I began to dance to the rhythm of the drum deep within, as I bonded to my roots through the study of my cultural heritage. I was transformed within and transfixed by cultural circles of spiritual freedom where I learned to love myself as an Afrakan born in America, a black woman, a woman of color. I healed my self-esteem by embracing my natural beauty; my hair, my lips, my nose, my hips, my skin. Nina Simone, Angela Davis, and Empress Akweke became my models of beauty. All of these circles helped birth me into a dancer, a drummer, a singer, an artist, a healer and a wellness warrior. The healer within me was reborn through every circle from age sixteen to sixty-one. Each circle that I entered had its way with me. Each circle molded me, purified me, formed me and pruned me; pulled me

(TRANSFORMATION)

up a bit higher than the round before. Each circle has given me greater inner vision and courage; sent me deeper into my inner center circle of oneness.

Look at the circle you are in. The way of the circle is that in this circle you are given the opportunity to live within a life-affirming circle or die in a circle of un-fulfillment. In the circle of life, remember that life is reflecting back to you as a mirror of your positive or negative self. Be courageous, look within and take responsibility for your life and what takes place within your circle. Be present in your conscious and subconscious state of mind. The circle is your creation. If your circle of life hurts, harms, belittles, stresses you then raise your frequency, detoxify your life and your circle will restore you. Pay close attention to your center circle, your path way to freedom. As each circle of consciousness brings one closer to oneself, layers of dead flesh and dead thoughts get left behind. Each circle comes with its own set of lessons. The lessons are about friends, family, work and love. All lessons, all circles grow you, give you back yourself.

• • • • •

As you journey from one circle maintain your center circle. The challenges will come and the harvest will come. Allow yourself to be transformed and you will overcome. "Go in and come to life." are words of power that were spoken for healing by our ancestors, ancient Wise Ones. Circles give us the tools to be the root and the rock, the feather and the flower; gathering from each circle the tools we need for liberation, joy, and harvest.

360°: THE PROCESS

Why use this guide: We begin life in the form of a circle; as a cell. Our whole body operates by using trillions of circles. Circles of blood cells oxygenate our blood stream. The tissues, organs and systems within our physical body are the intricate and divine functioning of circles. In like manner, circles are the pivotal element within, throughout and around our physical, emotional, financial and spiritual worlds. Whether you are aware of it not, you are constantly part of several circles, simultaneously. A circle of friends, a prayer circle, your family circle and all your relationships are the circles that make the circle of the self that you are. What you do in the Circle of Self determines the color and rhythm of your life. Remember what our parents told us, "Watch the company you keep in your circle." Your company is "you", if your company, your circle, is in disease and disarray then you will be in disease and disarray. On the other hand, if your company is positive, productive and on a path of wellness, then, you too will be positive, productive and on a path of wellness.

At any given time, you are a full circle, broken circle, unbroken circle; you are either drawn closer to or further away from feeling complete. When this feeling is positive and productive it is the engine/energy to wellness. When we are not fully oxygenated; we operate at 180 degrees, our circle is broken; we become stagnant and our circles become places of dysfunction and di-ease. When we are outside of a circle we feel isolated /lonely/ desperate. Circles are repeated cycles: good, bad and/or indifferent. The relationships we have to finances, food, health, politics and to other people comes from the circle into which we were born and raised, the Circle of Family; our primary circle.

We must begin at the beginning of our primary circle with an honest and healing awareness of self and with self in the family. We must acknowledge the presence of issues/elements that we carry year to year, circle to circle from our primary circle. We must identify and assess the relationships and the lessons. Determine to continue to support that which supports your wellness. We must notice the frequency of the occurrences of rejection, abandonment, disappointment and loss. Ask yourself: *How did I participate or was I a victim in the dysfunction?* Those behaviors which cause dis-ease must be changed and those relationships which cause dysfunction must be forgiven. Forgiveness offers release from the elements that cause dis-ease and that prevent healing, growth, and wellness. Forgiveness clears the ground for planting, cultivating and harvesting at 360 degrees.

How to use this guide: The worksheets in this guide are designed to assist you with the process of creating healthy, balanced, beautiful 360 degree circles.

Paradigm Shift 1:
Transformation contains specific exercise worksheets identified with an icon and the words: "Wellness Work." These worksheets focus on transforming your paradigm to consciously plant wellness in the body, mind, and spirit. The work begins with awareness of the Circle of Self as related to circles of your family, friends, mates, community and planet. Use worksheets in Paradigm Shift 1 to:

- become aware of Circle of Self
- recognize the circles in our life
- assess circles for confusion and balance
- recognize the lessons learned
- release /let go of pain and dis-ease
- forgive
- plant and cultivate specific circles in your life i.e.:
    - as caretakers for children
    - as caretakers for elders
    - as women
    - as men
    - as members of a community

Paradigm Shift 2:
Unification is an illustration of the union of holistic methods and allopathic medicine. Use this paradigm to examine the magnificent possibilities of circles united to plant, cultivate and harvest wellness.

The pages in Paradigm Shifts 3, 4 and 5 and Next Steps **are not identified** with an icon because all the pages provide information and guidance for your ongoing "Wellness Work" to plant, cultivate and harvest Circles of Wellness.

Paradigm Shift 3:
Restoration consists of strategies for using food as medicine to detoxify and purify.

Paradigm Shift 4:
Empowerment is predominantly instructions for using Wellness Tools. This chapter includes wellness self-assessment, and guides and illustrations of the 12 Empowerment Wheel Circles.

Paradigm Shift 5:
Rejuvenation is entirely wellness work with guides for creating a wellness home including appropriate affirmations, charts, and instructions to support preparation and usage of your home for Optimal Wellness.

The Earth circles the sun annually as it simultaneously circles around itself to face the sun, daily; circles upon circles. The sun creates a powerful frequency that has an impact on every living thing. When we tap into that frequency we create a chain reaction that will affect everyone in our circles. Our aim in life is to return to what our ancestors knew, and inherently what we know. We must aim to go back to the root of things: to eat off the land, to give generously; to perform full circle; to become 360 degrees, complete. When we operate within full circle frequency we will radiate abundance, fullness, evolution. As a complete Circle of Self we are constantly planting and cultivating new ideas. Fulfilment and success is the harvesting. If we plant and water healthy seeds, move through the seasons with balance, and cultivate and invest in wellness, we will harvest and benefit from our nourishing crop. Imagine a relationship, a family, a community or even a planet operating at 360 degrees. What mastery!

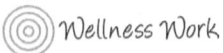 *Wellness Work*

CIRCLE OF AWARENESS

Become aware of relationships and lessons in the Circle of Self. Ask yourself: Which behaviors and relationships support my wellness? Next, ask yourself: Which behaviors and relationships have caused repeated dysfunction and dis-ease? Use this template to create your Circle of Awareness:

1. Place relationships inside these various sections in your circle. Include family members, friends, associates, partners and others who influence your life.
2. Write a name under each relationship. Next to the name write one word about how you feel about that person.
3. Write the lesson that each person has given.
4. Reflect on and acknowledge the lessons in order to evolve to freedom through overcoming.
5. Get busy breaking patterns of Emotional & Psychological Relationship Dis-Ease. Instead of imprisonment in anger and disappointment, use your past to promote your growth in wellness.
6. After reflection, write 1-3 words about how you feel about the lesson each person/relationship brought to your life.
7. If you cross off the names and relationships, you are left with the lessons. You will then notice the patterns and connections of the lessons that have been brought to you by your relationships. Reflect on the lessons so that the healing will be revealed to you. The lessons are given to you to help you develop awareness of the circles you are in and their state of confusion or balance with regard to your wellness of body, mind, finances, social relations and spirit. Once you are aware, you can take the appropriate next steps.

CIRCLES OF WELLNESS

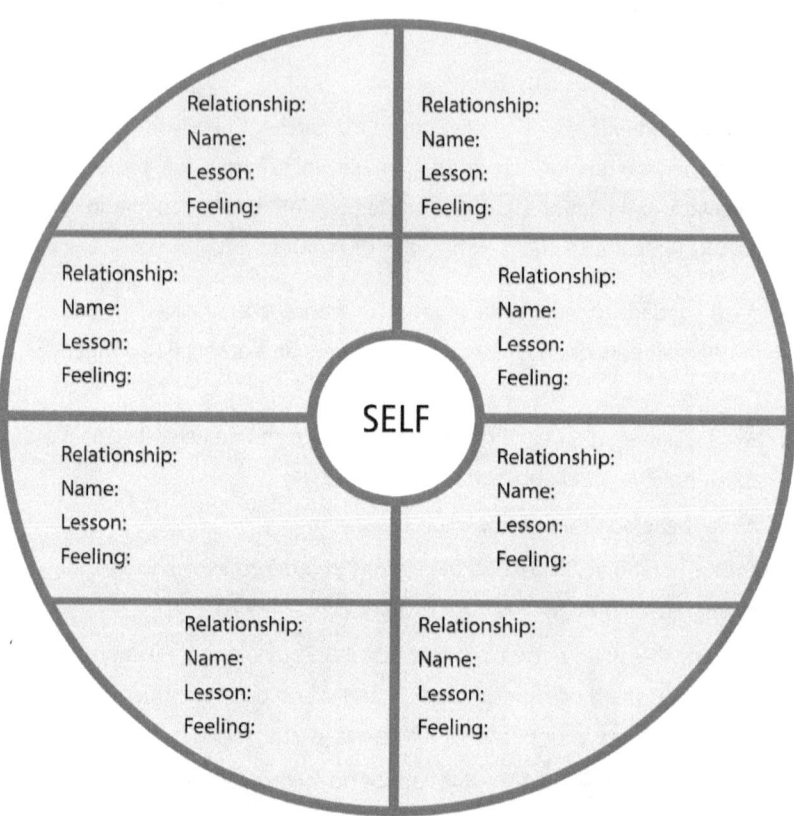

Every One Is My Teacher – Every Relation Is A Reflection of Self – Heal Yourself, Heal Your Relations

(TRANSFORMATION)

HOLISTIC LOVEMAKING

Calling all "Grown Folks", **this article is for you.** Calling all Spouses, Lovers, Sexual Partners, those *in* a sexual relationship, those *planning* to be in sexual relationship and those who *used to be* in sexual relationship, **this article is a must read.** I must tell you, that the Circle of Intimacy shared by you and your partner is everybody's business! So, for your sake and the sake of all of us, please: **Make Holistic Love, not toxic war.**

Recently, a growing number of my clients are declaring a sexual STATE OF EMERGENCY. Many of our young adults, the new "Grown Folks" are being **scared straight** by the increase of HPV (Human papillomavirus, the most common sexually transmitted infection in the United States.) and genital herpes infections which are running rampant in our communities at an alarming rate. Clients are calling and coming to see me, scared for their lives, feeling hopeless in the face of these devastating infectious diseases. Partners are passing diseases back and forth. Even if protection is worn during intercourse, toxic bodily fluids (wastes and poisons) usually transmitted by sexual organs, are being transmitted mouth to mouth and skin to skin, and then traveling throughout the bloodstream. So, who's really safe? The result of engaging toxicity during sexual relations can be compared to war causing war.

Partners not only have to deal with the physical effects of passing the infection to each other, but also with the psychological and emotional effects of blame and distrust. toxic lovemaking is the cause and result of unresolved psychological and emotional issues. Women and men are carrying "toxic baggage" into the bedroom. Hidden in the baggage are family dysfunctions from childhood, sexual abuse from past relationships, hit and run lovers, previous "down low" partners, self hate, fear, and more. Frequently, one or both partners are not even aware that the "baggage" exists. In this state of not knowing, the toxicity is magnified in each other's mental, emotional and physical being with each trust and each moan of pleasure. I recommend before engaging in sexual activity with a partner, please pause to reflect; think before you leap. You can avoid the regret;

you can avoid passing onto one another physical, psychological, emotional, or spiritual dis-ease, disharmony, and discomfort. Think, before you conceive a vision or a child who will be born into dis-ease caused by a disharmonizing exchange. Your thoughts and actions have an impact on all of your circles; and they have an impact on you. Too often those engaged in a Circle of Intimacy reflect negative models made popular through the music, social media and cyber exposure. We are bombarded with an attitude of disrespect and violence accepted not only as the norm, but also as the preferred behavior before, during and after the sexual act. We are saturated with the acceptance of this deteriorated social interaction, which greatly influences today's sexually active population. Indeed, this is a time of sexual STATE OF EMERGENCY.

DO NOT DESPAIR; KNOWLEDGE IS POWER.

It is time to make better choices. Learn to identify that which brings toxicity to your body, mind and spirit in the form of sexual activity, often disguised as lovemaking. If the behavior brings you harm; if it does not support your wellness then it is not making love, it is making war. Choose to DETOX immediately from dysfunction and dis-ease. Detox from the rage and from revenge. Men must stop calling women bitches. Women, that is not your name, stop answering to it. Shift away from unhealthy lifestyles; they do not support your wellness. Choose Holistic Living and Holistic Lovemaking for social change. Forgive. Shift your paradigm and expect to give and receive optimal pleasure and fulfillment during lovemaking. You can exude harmony and balance that will show up in every aspect of your life In addition, you can experience more powerful orgasms which will open you up to a more powerful, magnetic, energized life. **It does not happen in one day; it does take time.** Continue to use this guide book to plant, cultivate and harvest the circles in your life. You and your partner can begin by transforming your physical, emotional, mental, and spiritual wellness. Continue doing the "Wellness Work" on the following pages throughout this guide. Be Well.

(Transformation)

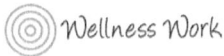 Wellness Work

Circle Of Intimacy

Change your lovemaking paradigm. You and your partner can create a wellness Circle of Intimacy and enjoy Holistic Lovemaking to the fullest. Overcome the causes of toxic lovemaking by completing more than one 21 Day Detox period. Continue on in your pursuit of Optimal Wellness by completing a full Detox Season (84 days).

Begin with your Circle of Self. Do your "Wellness Work" to become aware of the lessons.

Identify that which brings toxicity to your body, mind and spirit in the form of sexual activity.

Ask yourself: *Which behaviors support my wellness?* Make the paradigm shift to nurture wellness behaviors.

Ask yourself: *Which behaviors cause toxicity in my life?* DETOX immediately from dysfunction and dis-ease.

Determine with your partner whether your situation is mild or extreme. Together, establish a paradigm shift from unhealthy living to radiant, vibrant living.

Embrace: a detox lifestyle to restore your love relationships with yourself; to restore and prevent toxicity and aging of your sexual organs; to heal your relationship with your current partner. Apply for 21days if your situation is mild or up to 84 day if your situation is mild extreme.

Holistic Lovemaking Wellness Observances

Nutrition:

Avoid foods that cause bacteria to weaken your bloodstream and sexual organs.

Avoid foods that clog and weaken the arteries to your sexual organs. Prevention of a healthy blood flow to your organs denatures your organs. Eat fresh fruit, whole grain cereal. Use almond milk instead of cow's or goat's milk.

NO: flesh, dairy, fried foods, junk foods, inorganic foods, fast foods, GMO foods

Morning Meal (Tonics and Liquid meal):

Drink: Kidney liver flush: juice of two lemons/limes and 1 clove of garlic with 8 oz H2O

Drink: Green Life Nutritional Formula I with unsweetened cranberry juice 8-16 oz.

Additional vitamins and water: 100 mg of B-complex 3x a day, 500-1000 mg of vitamin C 3x a day; 25,000 IU of Vitamin E 1x a day; and 16 oz of H2O. 3x a day

For women: Woman's Life Herbal Formula –
For men: Man's Life Herbal Formula: Add 3 Tbs Herbal Formula to 3 cups of water, steep overnight, drink in morning.

Midday & Sunset: (Tonics and Liquid meal):

Drink: Green Life Nutritional Formula I with 8-12oz fresh green juice and 1-2oz fresh pressed wheatgrass

Additional vitamins: 50mg-100mg vitamin B complex/ 500-1000 mg of vitamin C/ 25,000 IV of vitamin 3

Midday & Sunset Meals (Solid Meal): Salads, steamed veggies, whole grain, veggie protein (ie beans, peas, raw soaked nuts, Eat okra 3x a week to detox the colon and your sexual organs.

Activities:

Create or Join a Forgiveness Circle

(TRANSFORMATION)

Do 10 minutes Inversion Therapy upon waking. Lay flat in bed. Place legs over three stacked pillows to send healing energy and oxygen and circulation into your sexual organs, your heart and your mind.

Perform a sweat 2-3x a week for 1 hour to flush bacteria out of your blood, skin and organs

Visit nature weekly at a botanical garden, park, ocean or daily in your backyard and/or garden

Exercise 3x a week: Power walking, Yoga, Tai-chi, Zumba, Dance (African, Brazilian, Haitian, Salsa)

Take an herbal laxative 2-3x a week for 21 days to promote elimination and thus remove pressure off of and bacteria out of your sexual organs

Have a colonic irrigation 2x a month to promote elimination and thus remove pressure off of and bacteria out of your sexual organs

Prepare a poultice of clay and gauze to apply overnight 3x a week. Women apply over your uterus. Men apply over your prostate.

Affirmation Work:

Affirm yourself upon raising daily and throughout your day. Claim that you are no longer a prisoner of dis-ease and that the power to heal is within.

Sexual Healing Technique: Perform the "Microcosmic" or the Rennenet Breath Meditation Circle to unblock and nourish the spiritual, physical, psychological and sexual body.

> Perform a sweeping inhalation breath, as you tighten your abs and anus. Breathe in and tighten from the navel, through the sexual organs up to the spine, to the first eye and crown. Perform several rounds raising up energy as you exhale and release your abs and anus.

Journal Work:

Write in your journal at sunrise and sunset. Release in writing the anger, pain, hurt, and disappointment of your past or present relationships. Log your progress.

To further your study on Holistic Lovemaking review my other books: *Heal Thyself for Health and Longevity* chapter 18 p. 197-208 and *Sacred Woman* Chapter 13 p.347. Also see: *Overcoming an Angry Vagina: Journey to Womb Wellness* and *Man Heal Thyself* for greater understanding of self and each other.

From Forgiveness To Freedom

The root of all dis-ease AND wellness is within the heart of EVERY man and of EVERY woman. The root of all dis-ease AND wellness is within the heart of YOU, husband, wife, father, mother, boyfriend, girlfriend, boss, co-worker, parent and child. Our unresolved hurt – wounded and broken hearts – cause the pain shaped as emptiness and hostility, revenge, and abuse. In our families and our communities, the pain and reaction to pain shows up as violence. On the global scale, the pain rages as war. Individually, around the globe our pain is the dis-eases we suffer in our hearts and our minds and throughout our bodies. Our unresolved hurt is depression and stress which travels through our nerves and blood as high blood pressure, sits in our colons as constipation, and locks our joints and bones with arthritis. Our unresolved hurt and pain in our broken heart is the root of confusion and disharmony in our relationships.

The Ancestral Wise Ones of the Nile Valley were acutely aware of the Power of the Heart to the point that they established the paradigm of justice, harmony and right living for the entire nation upon the heart and the importance of the heart being in balance with a feather on a scale. Thus, the term, "As light as a feather." The root of all wellness is within the heart of YOU, husband, wife, father, mother, boyfriend, girlfriend, boss, co-worker, parent and child. In order to heal ourselves and to restore ourselves to wholeness and peace, our hearts must be as light as a feather. We must seek to be balanced. We must detoxify the disharmony. We must forgive.

The Power to Heal is Within You. Do not give over your power to failure or illness. Take your power back, whether or not you think you are right. When your emotional self feels that your heart is broken, wounded and cut up into pieces, your physical self holds that depression and anxiety in your cells and nerves and muscles and organs and in your blood. That held in pain sets the stage for heart a attack and/or for a stroke. All the greatness that you have done in your life comes from within. All the challenges that you've experienced, comes from within. Forgiveness begins within you. First of all, forgive yourself.

Forgiveness creates purification; purification creates liberation. Hearts must be as light as a feather, daily, if we are to be whole. Our hearts must be clean and pure; free of anger and hatred and animosity and free of fear. For balance, health and healing we must be in a perpetual state of harmony and wellness (MAAT according to the ancient Wise Ones of the Nile Valley). The pathway to reach this elevated state is through forgiveness. You may ask, *"How do I forgive wrong acts done to me?"* You answer yourself, *"My mother did this, my father did that, my mate did this and my children did that"*. We have been wronged by family, friends and strangers. We have repeatedly experienced abandonment, fear, abuse, and loss. In our financial circle there has been loss, impoverishment, dissatisfaction and financial failure. There have been multiple dietary and wellness challenges, and on and on. To get free from the prison of pain in your body, mind, heart and spirit you must break the cycle; form new habits. Navigate your life from pain to freedom, one step at a time.

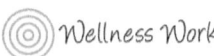

Wellness Work

Step 1
Look at your condition straight on. Take responsibility for its creation and existence. Realize that every experience that we live is the creation of our conscious and subconscious mind playing back to us our inner worries. Go into a quiet, still place in yourself. Breathe deeply into your heart center and ask the question: *"Why did it happen?"*

Step 2
Ask yourself, *"What is my lesson?"* As a student of life you receive the lessons that not only will free and heal you, but they also can be a healing balm for others. Every experience is a lesson for one to learn from and to grow through.

Step 3
Don't wait for someone to apologize, to ask for forgiveness or to take the first step. To transform is not about those who have done us wrong. It is about you making the paradigm shift to realize forgiveness within. Forgive everyone

fearlessly! As you do so, you will receive energy, hope and clarity to your life quest for well-being.

Step 4
Strive to become able to recognize that every lesson is a blessing; every experience makes you stronger in your thoughts, your actions and your state of being. Receive the lessons; learn from the lessons.

Step 5
And finally, give thanks for the clarity. Let the truth (MAAT) set you free and give you wings that you may fly to your most elevated, radiant, holistic self…and become as light as a feather.

*As you walk the road of forgiveness you walk the road of wellness.
Many deserved treasures await you for your efforts and hard work.
Continue to travel into the REBIRTH of your life.*

Daily Forgiveness Affirmation

I have the power to take responsibility for my life's journey.
I have the power to stand in my truth as a powerful mighty being
who makes the impossible, possible.
I have the power to listen from within,
and to be *in tuned* with my inner calling.
I have the power to learn from my life's lessons.
I will not hold animosity;
it does not support the growth of wellness.
Forgiveness is my pathway to freedom, my strength, my restoration
that will allow my heart and my soul to take flight.
Truth Lives.

After the collective recites the Daily Forgiveness Affirmation participants can share their heart challenges. Then burn sage or frankincense and myrrh in the circle as the collective repeats: "To forgive is to heal; to heal is to live."

(TRANSFORMATION)

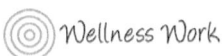 Wellness Work

ON THE WINGS OF FORGIVENESS

(A mirror meditation)
Woman, I invite you to break the cycle of pain
given one to another.
Man, I invite you to break the deadly cycle of pain
given one to another.
I know that each of you is hurt.
I invite you to speak. Come together;
face to face and heart to heart
to speak forgiveness for our recovery.
I invite us to speak so that we may forgive and love
and travel through our bloodline
to heal the past and the future.
I forgive you for the slaps and the kicks,
for the grabbing and the yanking,
for the shaking of my soul and my body.
I forgive you for the cursing
and the yelling and the screaming;
for the hostile words spoken,
 for the cruel tones and the harsh looks
that ruptured my veins
and traveled deep into my heart.

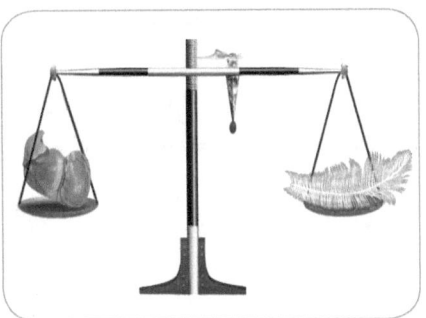

I forgive you for not keeping your word; your promise.
I forgive you for abandoning me, not being there
when I reached out.
I forgive you for not speaking gently,
when I needed comforting.
I forgive you for holding resentment towards me.
I forgive you for not knowing or understanding;
for not caring what I felt or how I felt.

I, woman, forgive you for being like my daddy,
or *not* being like my daddy.
I, man, forgive you for being like my mother,
or *not* being like my mother.
I want to overcome the pain that has filled my inner walls
with cancer, blood pressure, obesity and impotency.
I want peace and love; a new beginning.
Can we attract the beauty that is within me and you?
Will you forgive me whether I stay or move on;
whether I hold on or let go?

May we become wiser for the lessons we have learned?
May we hold in our hearts sweet, lasting forgiveness?
I forgive you for everything, as I forgive myself
for eating and covering up my pain
with dead thoughts and dead foods.
I forgive myself for living in a loop of unresolved wounds
of the heart, the spirit, the body & the mind.
I need soulful liberation.
I choose to be freed into the rapture of forgiveness.
I need to heal. I need my wings.
I forgive you. Will you forgive me? I forgive you.
Let us soar!

After the collective recites the Mirror Meditation participants can share their heart challenges. Then burn sage or frankincense and myrrh in the circle as the collective repeats: "To forgive is to heal, to heal is to live."

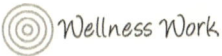 *Wellness Work*

GET OUT OF THE BOX

It is time to get out of the box and LET GO! Now that you have begun the paradigm shift away from blame and hurt toward forgiveness of yourself and of others, it is time to look at other blockages to your wellness. Taken one at a time, imagine that each blockage to your physical, mental and/or emotional well-being lingers in its own box while challenging your wellness, daily, weekly, yearly, and on into the decades of your life. You may be trapped in two, six, ten boxes at a time, all the time. each challenge dares you to escape. Use the reflections below to help identify the many boxes that could have you trapped. To effectively move into the power-filled Circle of Life you must, GET OUT OF THE BOX!

Part 1. Reflection

Reflection 1: Get Out of the Box
Are you in a box? Some boxes are so small that we can't move. Some boxes are filled with so much hurt that we can't breathe. Some boxes are wrapped with pretty paper, ribbons, bows and flower; but it's still a box. Inside your box are all the material things that you would want; nevertheless, it is still a box.

Reflection 2: Get Out of the Box
Are you living your authentic life? Is it your box, your mother's life, or your father's walk, or your mate's desires, or the social demands of your position, but not your life? Whose life are you living?

Reflection 3: Get Out of the Box
How do you know if you're in a box and not in a healing circle? A box contains you. A box surrounds you internally and externally with one or all of the following states of being that "box" you in with limitations. If you want to overcome states of limitation, get out of your box and come into a healing circle. Focus upon your Circle of Self.

Part 2. Focus Upon Your Circle Of Self. Identify States Of Limitation.

States of Limitation:

- Short sightedness
- Suppression
- Confusion
- Lack of confidence
- Entrapment
- Small thinking
- Shame
- Guilt
- Poverty
- Limited resources
- Toxic relationships
- Physical disease
- A wounded inner child
- Prostate and womb pain and trauma
- A revolving door of stress and anxiety
- A heavy heart
- Living somebody else's plan for your life

Journal and reflect on, "How did I get in the box of small thinking, toxic relationships or shame?" Then, get very still as you connect to your heart center. Look deeply as you ask, see and hear how you got into the box. Ask, "When", "Why", "How" and finally, "What" my life will be once I am out of the box. Write down your process in your journal so that you, now conscious, never return to the box again

(Transformation)

PART 3. Speak to yourself and plan your own personal liberation. Leap completely out of your box and affirm this daily at every sunrise and sunset so you can experience the wellness represented by the many States of Freedom. Radiate the "I AM greater" with each day:

States of Freedom:

- I am far sightedness
- I am a soul filled unity
- I am unlimited potential
- I am super-creative
- I am resourceful
- I am honesty
- I am confidence
- I claim healthy vibrant relationships
- I am unspeakably peace-filled
- I am purposeful with my work
- I am physically radiant
- I am mentally radiant
- I am spiritually radiant
- I release the past as I move forward
- I have the ability to help others get out of their box (es)

Be careful. Before you offer to align your life with another, at least start to get out of your box (es). Wait until you are sure you are free and will not fall back into the box. Continue, daily to cultivate and fortify your Circle of Freedom to support yourself before you seek to unify with and nurture others. Keep expanding into greater and more profound levels of freedom. If you ever find yourself in a box again – RUN, LEAP out of the box. Keep growing until there are no boxes in sight. Freedom is yours. Live it!

CIRCLES OF WELLNESS REFLECT CIRCLES OF LIFE

One way to look at our lives is through the lenses of circles. Observe the circles below that represent the constant and simultaneous flow of the aspects of our lives.

It is not possible to eat continuously without rest and digestion of food. There is no day without night; nor sunrise without sunset. To fully heal yourself and sustain wellness you must extend wellness to others; *this* is how we complete our wellness cycle. We must form or become a part of a Wellness Circle. The Circles of Wellness should strive to reflect the naturalness of the Circles in Life. Our wellness goals should include balance, completeness, fullness, activation and manifestation.

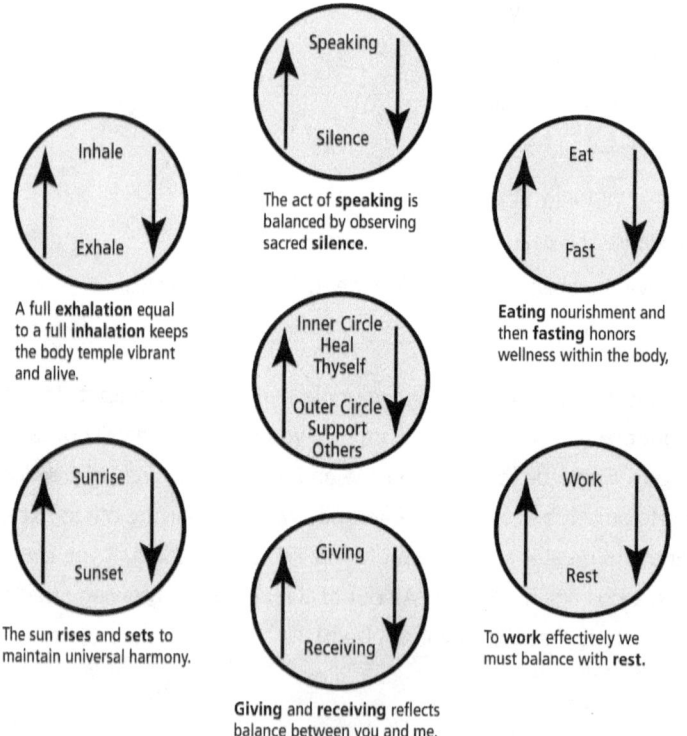

A full **exhalation** equal to a full **inhalation** keeps the body temple vibrant and alive.

The act of **speaking** is balanced by observing sacred **silence**.

Eating nourishment and then **fasting** honors wellness within the body.

The sun **rises** and **sets** to maintain universal harmony.

Giving and **receiving** reflects balance between you and me.

To **work** effectively we must balance with **rest**.

(Transformation)

Heal Your Life. Form Healing Circles.

Form a Healing circle. Come into a Healing circle. Make a paradigm shift right now. It is time to transform. In order to grow, to transform, and to heal chose one or more: A Drum Circle. A Dance Circle. A Prayer Circle. A Meditation Circle. A Healing Circle. A Spiritual Circle. A Support Circle. An Economic Circle. A Womb Wellness Circle. A Fitness Circle. A Man Heal Thyself Circle. A Sacred Woman Circle. A New or Full Moon Circle. A Child Care Circle. A Study Group Circle. A Medicine Circle. A Sweat Lodge Circle. Form a Circle of Light or a Circle of Hope. Come into a Circle of Growth or a Circle of Peace.

Circles are cultural, magical, redeeming, fulfilling and inspirational. Circles immediately transform us from being isolated, closed off and shut in, to being opened, connected, unified and compassionate. Circles make easy the bonding of heart to heart and soul to soul. In circles we touch, we see, we share in love our differences and our common grounds. In circles we open up, we listen, we forgive. In circles we tune up like a violin, a harp, a drum to harmonize, effortlessly. We become one with nature (Air, Fire, Water, Earth). We synchronize.

Some may have been wounded in circles and say "I will never be in circle again." However, Life is a circle! How do you stop living while being? The more in tune you are, the healthier your circles will be. Your circle reflects and radiates who you are and what you are seeking. Your circle reflects your frequency of vibration. If you are challenged within the circle, but you know the circle is right for you – go deeper. Allow the circle to purify you, to restore you, no matter what reflections come up. Remember, "The power to heal is within you. You have the power to heal yourself." Take responsibility for your part in the circle. Take responsibility for the circle of your creation. Metaphorically speaking, while you are in the eye of the hurricane (those challenges that the circle brings), you are being cleansed. In the midst of the fire the flames are burning away mental, emotional and physical disease. Inside the circle are your lessons. Embrace them and soar to your highest self. Just as the caterpillar becomes the butterfly, you are transforming to the beauty of your complete circle self. Continue chanting:

CIRCLES OF WELLNESS

"The power to heal is within me...I have the power to heal myself."

Healing Circles can offer us refuge and be safe havens of peace. At 2 o'clock in the morning while completing notes for this text, I was in a Circle of Channeling with a devotee of healing, Quasheba, who shared with me that a circle should protect. She noted that her life "...feels protected when in circles, traveling from port to port, from one circle of healing into another." Be wise in your circling; stay in tune. Know when it is time to stay in a circle and when it is time to leave one circle and enter into another.

Circles bond us, liberate us and uplift us. Recognize your Circle of Self. Form circles in small or large groups. You will heal just by being within one. Healing Circles give off a frequency of light, of beauty, of sacredness, of spiritual majesty and of Divine Power. Circles help us to grow, to prosper and to live in harmony with life. At every opportunity create a circle with friends, family, strangers, youth and the elderly. Join with women, with men, with wise people and with people new in our lives. Find your circles on the Internet, through social media, in your school or spiritual center, at home or within your community. Make circling a daily practice for our collective liberation, as we focus on healing the planet from discord and from disease. We each have automatic permission to liberate ourselves. As we form circles and come into circles around the planet, we will be closer to Global Healing.

(Transformation)

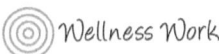 Wellness Work

REJUVENATE YOUR COMMUNITY

Dear Seeker of Wellness and Peace,

Please be advised that it is always a good time to rejuvenate. If you are seeking to get better yourself, then joining with others may provide the support. Meanwhile, if you are satisfied with the progress you are making on your wellness, your energy may be just what is needed in a circle of family or friends or colleagues. Think community. Do circles.

Step 1
Become a conscious Citizen of Wellness. Participate in the seasonal One Day Detox Program and/or join the 21 Day Detox Program.

Step 2
Form/join a Circle of Wellness with others who are ready to "heal thyself". Use the Circle of Wellness CD Empowerment Series and the instructions in this text to aid you on your journey to the City of Wellness. As an evolving citizen of wellness, reach out to family, friends and associates.

Step 3
"Each One, Teach One". Each person of an initial circle is responsible for spreading wellness by starting new Circles of Wellness.

Step 4
Follow a season (84 days). Replicate Steps 2 and 3.

Step 5
Stay in touch. Participants in Circles of Wellness should meet weekly to support self and group wholeness.

Who can form Circles of Wellness?

- Spiritual Leaders
- Doctors
- Housewives
- Artists
- Lawyers
- Wellness Practitioners
- Politicians
- Book Club Leaders
- Teachers
- Community Activists
- Service Providers
- Radio And Television Personalities
- Managers
- All Concerned Citizens
- YOU!

WE ALL CAN MAKE A WELLNESS DIFFERENCE!!!

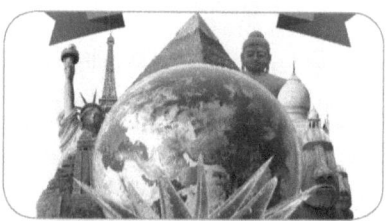

When can I form Circles of Wellness?

Right now, Reach out, your circle is waiting.

(TRANSFORMATION)

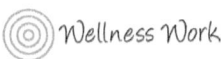 Wellness Work

HOW TO PLANT CIRCLES OF WELLNESS

As one in your own Circle of Wellness, it is your mission to bring four more people into your circle. Write down the names of "your people". Think of those at home, in the neighborhood, at school and/or your place of worship. Now, chose the top four who you feel will join you on your journey. CALL THEM! Invite them to join your Circle of Wellness for the opportunity to create a NEW SELF and a NEW COMMUNITY of wellness.

As with every gathering, not everyone who is invited shows up. So, put extra people on your list. Begin here and now listing people to invite to your Circle of Wellness.

Name	Contact	Numbers

1. _____

2. _____

3. _____

4. _____

5. _____

6. _____

7. _____

8. _____

9. _____

10. _____

Make notes for scheduling and for planning your circle agenda:

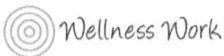 Wellness Work

How To Cultivate Circles Of Wellness

A Global Circle of Wellness weekly support meeting is a holistic workshop. Global Circles of Wellness begin with a single seed. You are the one that has been chosen to grow into wellness and then share your growth with others in need of healing. As a seed, you will flower and contribute to building the community by helping others to flower. You must be willing to reach out to others and encourage them to grow into their wholeness. As a seed you make the commitment to meet weekly, monthly or seasonally to uplift humanity into global healing. Once you have established a Circle of Wellness follow the steps in the AGENDA FOR CIRCLE MEETINGS article and the suggestions bellow.

Gather for one to three hours to share wellness information and inspire one another with empowering healing testimonies.

Partake in an herbal tea ceremony. Share the herbal blend presented in the 12 Empowerment Wheel Circles of Chapter 4 or the Master Herbal from the 21 Day Detox Kit.

Read and discuss topics from appropriate texts. The reference texts should include **Heal Thyself for Health & Longevity** and **The City of Wellness: Restoring Your Health Through the 7 Kitchens of Consciousness** by Queen Afua. The circle should be open to the introduction of other holistic books that could further grow the collective consciousness.

Have a once a month potluck meal at your Circle of Wellness meeting. You might choose to enjoy luscious vegetarian recipes found in *The City of Wellness* by Queen Afua or other texts that provide vegetarian and vegan-friendly recipes.

Invite others to join our Circles of Wellness. The once a month potluck meal provides an excellent opportunity to introduce individuals and families in the

CIRCLES OF WELLNESS

community to the benefits and joys of a holistic lifestyle, this is a grassroots way of planting seeds. This is how we can grow a powerful wellness movement.

Notice a paradigm shift. When you form a Circle of Wellness, each of you will notice a shift in your own life and in the lives of those in your circle. You can bear witness to and make an impact on a global shift from toxicity toward wellness.

Join Our Monthly Circle of Wellness 21 Day Detox Program

AFFIRM: "In my inner circle, I affirm wellness. In my family circle, I affirm wellness. In my circle of friends, I affirm wellness.

Among my associates, neighbors, staff, co-workers, I affirm wellness. There is wellness in my circle."

Make notes for follow-up activities:

_____

_____

_____

_____

_____

_____

_____

_____

_____

_____

_____

(Transformation)

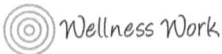 Wellness Work

Agenda For Circle Meetings

(The following is a suggested outline for weekly meetings. It is important to include all the steps. Eventually your meeting will develop its own rhythm.)

- **Open** the session with the Circle of Wellness Daily Affirmation.
- **Conduct** a 2 to 5 minute meditation with breathing exercises.
- **Focus** on the harmony in the Circles of Wellness and Circles of Life.
- **Drink** Master Herbal Formula II Tea or an herbal tea that complements for this week's goal.
- **Introduce** yourselves and express your interest in maintaining a united circle. New invitees share their desire for seeking to join the circle.
- **Share** experiences from the previous week. This could be a challenge, a breakthrough of feelings about new endeavors such as aerobics, yoga, power walking and so forth...
- **Agree** on a **collective goal** and purpose for choosing *that* goal for next week. The goal could be to release using sugar or to meditate for five minutes three days next week and so forth.
- **Document** the selection in your journals. The tea for next week's meeting should compliment next week's goal and can be selected at this point.
- **Review and discuss:** "9 STEPS TO WELLNESS EMPOWERMENT and HOLISTIC LIVING" (See Paradigm Shift 3).
- **Select** one member to "testify" about the benefits of holistic lifestyle living to their wellness.
- **Close** the meeting with the Circle of Wellness Daily Affirmation.
- **Prepare and enjoy** a Circle of Wellness Potluck Meal once a month. Participants should contribute a potluck dish (food or beverage) from a recipe found in: *The City of Wellness: Restoring Your Health Through the*

7 Kitchens of Consciousness by Queen Afua or other texts that provide vegetarian and vegan friendly recipes.

AFFIRM: "I establish and bring forth wellness in my circle, as I affirm to do my part of lifting up all my relations. Hands On, Hands Out, Hands Around the World; Our World."

Make notes for follow-up activities:

_____

_____

_____

_____

_____

_____

_____

_____

_____

_____

_____

_____

_____

_____

(Transformation)

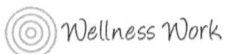 Wellness Work

INNER CIRCLE MEDITATION

All circles reflect your own relationship to self. Support your circle as it takes you onto higher ground and gives you optimal wellness. Perform an inner circle meditation every sunrise and sunset.

Sit still in a cross-legged position or sit comfortably in a chair, place palms upward in your lap.

Relax and center your body, mind and spirit to your breath.

Breathe a circular breath of peace (Hotep). Then as a circle of breath and light, breathe in and out through your nostrils as you expand your inner circle.

Perform this circle of breath and light with each breath as your inner circle becomes more radiant, more electric and more alive within you.

Allow this circle to flow several times until you feel the presence of the oneness within your Body, Mind and Spirit.

Be still.

Be an open vessel for your inner circle to vibrate through every part of your being as you feel the love, the calm, the protection the fullness of your inner circle.

Empower your circle.

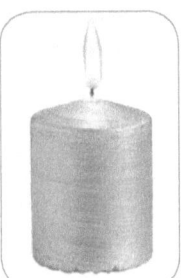

Offer this Inner Circle Meditation process to your inner Divinity for peace and harmony.

The harmony that you establish within
will follow you into any circle along your path.

Make It A Million

The City of Wellness Master Plan to Global Wellness

Begin your journey to wellness by joining our Circle of Wellness
Follow Queen Afua's all natural
21-Day Detox & Purification Health Program
Become educated on how to expand your circle
into a potential network of one million-plus people

ONE MILLION PLUS

Month	People
8th Month	1,578,400
7th Month	409,600
6th Month	102,400
5th Month	25,600
4th Month	6,400
3rd Month	1,600
2nd Month	400
1st Month	100

Growth is determined by each member starting a circle of 4
upon completion of their 21-Day Program

Get on board
transform your City of Wellness
into ONE MILLION-PLUS strong

Create New Families
Create New Communities

(TRANSFORMATION)

THE PEOPLE HAVE THE POWER

The power to heal and restore your wellness is in your hands and hearts. As we, "Each one teach one", we become wellness circles of change. Circles of Wellness on fire with wellness fire become inspired to help family and friends. As Circles of Wellness grow within and around us, the City of Wellness grows. Our efforts will raise humanity to wholeness of body, mind and spirit. We all have the power to heal ourselves, our relations and our relationships. We do not have to live with disease; we can learn how to live with wellness.

One Vision
The City of Wellness will encourage citizens to join the path to wellness. The goal of each City of Wellness citizen (a Circle of Wellness unto herself/himself) is to inspire at least 100 people to be the seed to become an individual Circle and then host more circles of family and friends. An individual Circle of Wellness Green Seed Host is a wellness activist who, as the first healer in the home serves as the spark to inspire friends and families to heal themselves. Become a Circle of Wellness facilitator by gathering four people to perform wellness activities. This will help to grow our family into wellness and vitality. This helps to ensure their personal success; we are the company we keep. Each of the four should gather four more friends and family members who then become sixteen. Each of the sixteen should gather four people who will become sixty four. From the original Green Seed Hosts, the 100 become 400. The individual Circles of Wellness multiply into teams which eventually become one million-plus strong citizens in the Global City of Wellness. All those in the circle gather at the root for Circle of Wellness trainings, formulas and support at the Queen Afua Wellness Center.

In Time
One season is 84 days; two seasons is 168 days, 8 months and so on. Circles should continue to meet and grow over a full season. Wherever there are Circles of Wellness and a City of Wellness Home Team, there is the opportunity for a collective wellness vision to be established. We can change our environments

for the better. We can influence creating healthier soil for planting healthier trees and plants. We can focus on rejuvenating the environment so that we have more purified air to breathe and more purified water to drink. With these changes we, the people, can regenerate as well. The result can be vibrant, loving, alive citizens overcoming body, mind and spiritual disease. The cities can become healthier. The people can become empowered; wellness, rather than disease and disharmony can spread. There can be one million plus wellness citizens in each city. Cities of Wellness cannot be stopped nor blocked; north, south, east, or west, in every direction you turn there can be wellness. In time.

Right Now
Right now, civic leaders, teachers, lawyers, mothers, fathers, accountants, service providers, artists, we the people are becoming citizens of wellness. Crime is going down, wellness is on the rise! Statistics on disease are decreasing; wellness is on the rise! Employment is increasing because the people have unleashed their creative genius and are realizing their work. The City of Wellness is on the rise! Violence is decreasing; religious wars are lessening. Wellness is on the rise and is spreading like a blaze. We are growing in numbers, as brilliant vibrant Cities of Wellness.

WELLNESS IS ON THE RISE!

(TRANSFORMATION)

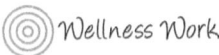 Wellness Work

WOMB WELLNESS CIRCLES

Who should form Womb Wellness Circles?
If a woman has a stressed out womb *or* a happy womb; if her womb has been beaten down *or* lifted up, a Womb Wellness Circle is for her. Women suffering with fibroid tumors or who have had a hysterectomy, a Womb Wellness Circle is for you. Sisters, mothers, daughters, from the four directions of the globe should form Womb Wellness Circles in order to heal yourselves and your relations.

Who is a Womb Circle Gatherer?
A Womb Circle Gatherer has a big heart and a willing spirit. She brings women together to heal themselves. She creates a safe haven of confidentiality where heart and soul sharing is encouraged and supported. She understands the relationship of the wellness of the physical womb to the wellness of the mind, heart and body. A Womb Circle Gatherer follows the philosophy, "Each one, teach one" on the journey towards personal wellness and peace on Earth. She is inspired from within. She may be you.

How do we set the tone for a Womb Wellness Circle Gathering?
A circle symbolizes opening the heart to heal – to forgive – to love again. Once a group of women has formed their circle, look for a space (in someone's home or in a community center). Purify the space: wash the floors with natural cleansers and smudge the area with sage or frankincense and myrrh. Arrange seating (chairs or beautiful pillows) in a circle. Set a candle on a cloth as a meditation focal point. Light the candle. Color suggestions for the cloth and the candle: White – purification and cleansing; Blue – peace and serenity; Pink – love and forgiveness; Lavender – elevation of the spirit. *Love Note: If a woman in your group is surviving from a womb trauma, such as a hysterectomy or a miscarriage or rape, consider dedicating the Circle Gathering to her healing.*

How do we conduct a Womb Wellness Circle Gathering?

After lighting the candle, read the Womb Awakening Affirmation (see below) to begin overcoming womb challenges. Visualize for a few moments life affirming womb wellness. See yourself birthing yourself away from pain and anger, into a healthy womb of peace and balance. Place your palms over your "first eye" in the center of your forehead and recite, "I bless the womb of my mind; what I think, I create." Breathe in and out, deeply. Next, place palms over your heart and recite, "I bless the womb of my heart; what I feel, I create". Breathe in and out, deeply. Now, place palms over your physical womb area and recite, "I bless the womb of my reproductive center; what I think and feel I birth in my womb center." Again, breathe deeply. Give thanks for the unification of the wombs of your mind, your heart and your reproductive center.

How do I connect to my Inner Voice of the Womb?

Be quiet and listen to you inner voice. Deeply breathe 28 rapid fire breaths for alignment. Close your eyes and go within; trust your intuition. Communicate with your inner voice. Upon receiving your messages for healing, write in your journal. Share your journal entries within the Womb Wellness Circle.

How do we share our Womb Stories?

Trust yourself to share your story. Open up, breathe deeply. Heal your heart; release the burdens, flush out the pain. Nurture your soul to wellness. Sisters' stories will heal sisters. Write in your journals again. You are on the threshold of a new beginning.

How do we close our circle gathering?

Embrace your sisters in gratitude. The Womb Circle Gatherer serves Woman's Life Herbal Formula or a soothing herbal tea. Enjoy the tea as it calms your body and soul. End the gathering by reciting a meditation or the Womb Awakening Affirmation. Before separating the group should schedule their next meeting place and date.

Suggested gathering times: During the new moon (beginning); during the full moon (rebirthing); once every 28 days. For deep womb wellness work it is recommended that the circle gathers weekly over a season (84 days).

What tools should I gather for my Womb Wellness Self Care?
Support your womb work by joining a Womb Wellness Circle and using womb wellness products. (Suggested products: 21 Day Detox Kit, Nutrition Kitchen Chart, Womb Yoga Chart).

What is my Womb Wellness homework?
Perform womb work throughout a season (84 days). Eat holistically. Journal daily. Bathe and self massage at least 3x a week. Love yourself unconditionally. Birth your purpose. Perform Womb Yoga every sunrise and sunset. Read material that supports your nurturing, recovery, purification and serenity. Encourage and witness your inner and outer transformation...until we meet again....

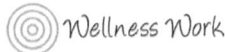
Wellness Work

WOMB AWAKENING AFFIRMATION

I have awakened to Womb Wisdom.
I have stretched my heart and my soul to the universe,
crying out for a womb healing...
my prayer has been answered; my consciousness has awakened,
so I bless in advance the rebirth of my Lotus-like womb.
As I journey deep inside myself to discover the secret healing of the Lotus;
I find a seed, the Lotus seed of illumination that so sweetly dwells
in the mist of the mud, within me.
This is a place where my lessons and trials reside.
This is the beginning of my womb healing; my womb awakening.

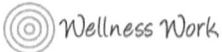 *Wellness Work*

MEN, FORM YOUR CIRCLES

Men it is time to form your circles! Yes, **YOU,** Business Man, Cultural Man, Spiritualist and Health Activist Man.

Dare to seek wellness solutions through consultation, products, workshops and seminars.

- **Walk** together.
- **Run** together.
- **Exercise** together.
- **Talk** together.
- **Prepare food and eat together.**
- **Trust** a brother.
- **Meditate/pray and be still** in a brotherhood circle.
- **Study and discuss solutions** together.
- **Support each other** in your quest for wellness.
- **Support each other** to stop the consumption of dead flesh that leads to dis-ease and a shortened life expectancy.
- **Teach each other** the responsibilities and rewards of a holistic life that honors and protects the family and the planet.

Come on, Brother from 'Around the Way' Man, claim your wellness. It is 'busting down the door' time. **Wellness Warrior Men,** form circles to **encourage** those making the shift to get off the drugs, cigarettes, and alcohol poisoning their blood and stifling their thinking. Come on, **Wellness Warrior continue** to **transform** yourselves and then reach out to assist others on their quest to take back their lives.

(TRANSFORMATION)

The Wellness Warrior fights to overcome a toxic lifestyle. He engages in **detoxification** and rejuvenation techniques, daily. He protects himself from falling prey to toxicity of drugs, alcohol and tobacco. He **strives to eliminate** flesh food, junk food and micro-waved food from his food plan. He **transforms** himself as Malcolm X said, "…by any means necessary." **stand shoulder to shoulder** with your Wellness Warrior brothers. **Fortify** each other to become an army of Healing Juggernauts.

Gather your resources, Juggernaut Men. Form circles to **rescue** the men on the vicious over-the-counter drugs cycle. Support the men striving to escape from taking over-the-counter drugs for temporary relief of toxic symptoms, to the need for more potent substances to numb the pain because temporary relief drugs wear off. Often the more potent substances are other OTC drugs, illegal drugs, toxic food and toxic sexual encounters. Still, the hurt doesn't go away; the vicious cycle continues. **Form circles** with the men who are ready to get rid of 'the monkey' on their back.

Be diligent, Holistic Medicine Men from the four directions. Walk in the footprints of the elders and ancestors to help the man in the midst of body, mind, spiritual, and relationship disparity. **Study the work** of those who held their ground and paid their dues in order to become master healers. **Be encouraged to encourage** men who have been suffering for generations. The chains of dis-ease and disharmony have disabled men (and their families) from past days of plantation slavery to the present days of prison-industrial slavery. We call upon all men to **join circles** and **become empowered** to break the chains that have destroyed lives in the form of poor dietary habits and dis-eases of body, mind and spirit.

Wellness Warriors, you not only will defend your right to live a healthy vibrant life, but you also fight for the restoration and rejuvenation of your family, friends, associates and community. You are a warrior for the global population's right to wellness. Circle after circle, Wellness Warriors and Healing Juggernauts **share the path of wellness** with the multitude. Salute to these men who have been on the front lines devoted to wellness work for decades and scores.

(CIRCLES OF WELLNESS)

Master Healers, Brothers, Fathers, Elders, Men of Wellness, form circles and continue to **hold tight to your wellness** convictions. Dare to become the living legacy of great, mighty, wise men. Continue to use the elements to create packs and wraps and to smudge, and to sweat and to eat natural, whole foods and herbs. Continue to teach each other how to liberate with wellness yourselves and the children you produce. Within you are the seeds of tomorrow. You are the physical, mental, emotional and social parents of the generations to follow. Men, **prepare yourselves** in circles of wellness. Let us look forward to the birth of well babies, who as returning giants can save humanity.

Men, become a Wellness Warrior, a Healing Juggernaut; a force to be reckoned with in your defense of wellness. Your battle tools are determination, commitment and conviction. It takes your full force and your convictions to break the cycle of toxic mental, physical, sexual and dietary addictions. It takes your full attention to tap into your inner wholeness. The Wellness Warrior Man aims to become **enlightened** and whole in body, mind, and **spirit.** The Wellness Warrior Man is **YOU** diligently on your path to wellness!

(Transformation)

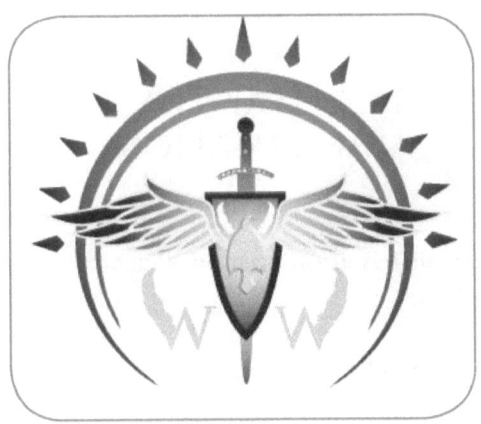

The Wellness Warrior Shield

The Wellness Warrior Protective Shield contains:
The feather of Maát
represents balance, truth and justice.
The sword of Bes
represents cutting away corruptible matter
to move beyond limitations.
The Falcon, king of the air
soaring above adversity
represents leadership and self mastery,
The surrounding circle
represents a continuum of eternal power.

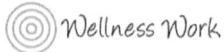 Wellness Work

MAN HEAL THYSELF AFFIRMATION

Below is the **Man Heal Thyself Affirmation,** as quoted from the Papyrus of Ani from Ancient Kemet.

Men, recite these words with conviction.

Men, recite these words with personal commitment.

Men, recite these words in the company of other men on the path to Optimal Wellness.

"May I open my two eyes which are blind.
May I stretch out my feet which are fastened together.
May my legs be strong and raise me up.
I know my heart,
I have gained power over my hands and arms.
I have gained power over my two feet.
I have gained the power to do what pleaseth my soul.
May my soul and body not be imprisoned.
I rise and shine...
I am powerful, I am mighty,
I come forth in peace".

from The Papyrus of Ani
(Transliteration and Translation by E.A. Wallis Budge)

(Transformation)

Save Our Children

This message is **"WELLNESS WORK" for all. It is a call out** to the caretakers of our children. Parents, godparents, grandparents, aunts and uncles, and teachers:

Circle around our children to heal and protect them.
As a person of African heritage born and raised in America, as a parent, I feel profound concerns. The extreme high rate of the murder of our sons and daughters is tragic. The incidence of suicides committed by our teenagers is tragic. As a Holistic Practitioner, I know Wellness Instructions are in order. As a Holistic Practitioner, I share with love, some ways to detox, preserve and restore our children.

Death By Murder

I SEE/WE SEE:
This message is in honor of four little Black girls, our daughters who were murdered while in church, a bomb meant to kill, and did. No more ribbons and bows, no more pretty dresses. No more A+ on school grades; hopscotch and jump rope; and hugs from loved ones. Murdered in Alabama -- in my father's home town in the Deep South. This message is because in Staten Island, New York and Ferguson, Missouri our sons gunned down by the police officers, hired to protect our lives... again. "War on terror" has come home ...police in riot gear disperse the crowd...war on our sons and daughters... ...unfair to people of color...again...and again...

WE RISE:
We the people must rise up against these atrocities. We the parents, the family, the caretakers, the communities must circle around all of our children and begin to create healing homes, safe havens, and detox sanctuaries, where we can raise our children. We must charge them with vibrant, loving, holistic action that will be a powerful "parent shield" of protection.

Death By Suicide

I SEE/WE SEE:

Our children are crying out for help. They are suffering to the point of death. Our children are our treasure; they represent the future, our hope, our potential and possibilities. Our children are suffering from depression, Bipolar Disorder, anxiety, hopelessness, distress from broken families. Some children suffer from sexual abuse, some are raised as "lone soldiers"-- "latch key" kids—going home alone to a no adult supervision or care. Some are from wounded parents who pass their hurt and wounded DNA down to their children. Some children suffer from a family setting of violence and drug and alcohol abuse. Some children are suffering from nutritional deficiency (malnourishment) to the brain, the nervous system and the blood. With the rise of technology, many of our youth suffer from cyber-bullying which is children murdering other children's self esteem and self-worth at the child's core and heart and soul.

WE RISE:

There must be a healing.

Caretakers Must Heal

If the parents are addicted to drugs and alcohol the child may be subject to verbal and physical and sexual abuse. In order to save our children in the home the parents and the caretakers should rejuvenate themselves with Green Life Formula I to balance and fortify mental and physical health. They should take Master Herbal Formula II to detox the body. They should strive to live a natural lifestyle based on a flexitarian or vegetarian or vegan diet or raw food. The child does not fall far from the tree that is the parent. As parents and caretakers heal, so, too, the children will heal.

Become Healers of Our Homes

Caretakers, parents: We are Healers of our home and of our lives and of our children, and we can heal ourselves and all of our relationships; for all our relationships are our reflections. As we the parents and grandparents, aunts and uncles heal ourselves, we heal our children. To protect your children as a caretaker your must live a Holistic lifestyle. In order to detox the body, mind, spirit and emotions and economies of the family, take yourself and your children through a 21 Day to 12 week Circle of Wellness Detox process.

Family, Circle Around Our Youth
Circles help to protect our children. Families form circles around your children in word, thought and deed. Caretakers fortify your children daily. Cultivate their talents. Communicate with your youth who are seeking positive values. Encourage them; support their visions. Help them to set up their business sooner rather than later. Build their entrepreneurial skills no matter how young. Feed them words that will form great character and create a powerful force field around them to protect them. Strengthen their force field by pouring empowering words into their minds. Build high self-esteem by educating your child on the greatness of their history.

Empowering Our Teens to Learn to Heal Thyself
As your child goes forth in the world if they are fully empowered by their caretakers, they can be protected from being discouraged by media, "frienemies" or ill-meaning peers. If the family circle at home is cultivated in strength and support, media-bullying will not be able to destroy them. Negativity will bounce off of children/teens who are charged, illuminated and functioning at high frequency. Offset the negativity that bombards our children in the form of racism by speaking to your child of the greatness of their race and the champions in their bloodline. Tell them they come from survivors who have overcome insurmountable odds and that greatness is within them. Your child will go into the world empowered and protected. Encourage teens to be healers.

I was invited to participate in a Holistic Panel to support high school students in their projects. The project was developed by the Future Project Dream Directors of New Jersey of which my son Supa Nova Slom Hip-Hop Medicine Man is a Dream Director. I listened to twelve groups of teenagers from various cities and schools share their stories. Seven out of twelve groups revealed that a friend, a classmate, a family member had committed suicide. I was shocked at the state of our children.

Seven out of twelve groups dedicated their projects to the classmates who had taken their lives. In one presentation after the next the teens spoke up for their friends. These youth, unified through the guidance of the Dream Directors, had formed Circles of Healing to create legacies of healing instead of sad remnants of broken souls. The children rose up and became leaders to aid other youth in harm's way. Maybe these conscious teens will catch a teen and prevent a suicide in the making. Maybe they will help a teen Heal Thyself just by caring enough to reach out.

Break the Chains
As a parent and caretaker, remember that as well as the good things of your life, unfortunately the negative aspects -- your pain, unresolved issues, past hurts, resentment, and hostility-- also pour out from you into your child's mind, body and spirit. This becomes a never-ending influence of negative pathologies that our children internalize as well as attract. Although the following is a report regarding the gang population in our communities, the message is absolutely for all members of the community.

About five years ago my eldest son, Supa Nova Slom, his brother Ali Amenche and the Wellness Warriors under "Heal the Hood" banner brought together from around the community over 300 teens and young adults who were gang members of the Crips and the Bloods. They gathered at our community center, Smai Tawi/Heal Thyself/ Know Thyself, to participate in a conference to end violence among our youth. Also invited was the leader of the Bloods who gave a powerful keynote address to the youth about the urgency to stop the killing and to put down their guns against one another. After his keynote mandate, he further counseled many of the most challenged youth who previously had murdered a fellow teen on the "battlefield" of the streets. At that event Supa Nova Slom had various members of the Crips and Bloods read aloud from the ***Willie Lynch Letter: The Making of a Slave.*** In the letter, written in 1712 Willie Lynch advises fellow owners of enslaved Africans of the necessity to "...divide in order to conquer the slaves." He guarantees that this tactic ensures that "slaves will stay as slaves for generations to come."

Transformation

Over 300 years ago, Willie Lynch told those who wanted to maintain control over the enslaved Africans that they must first control their minds and wills by ensuring that the "slaves" distrust each other over basic differences: age, skin color (complexion), hair texture, intelligence, size, gender, and status (house or field slave). Distrust and the "in-family" crimes that have followed has been the strongest link in the chains holding back liberation for over 300 years. It is past time to break the chains in order to heal.

First and last, there is no time to waste blaming. We have the power to heal our lives. Concentrate on recovery and restoration. Remember, words have power. Negative words had the power to cause distrust within the "family" and to psychologically enslave generation after generation. Positive words supported with a mighty force of positive holistic living must be employed to reverse 300 years of damage and lay the foundation for circles of wellness in the families and in the communities.

Affirm daily: "No more violence upon our sons and daughters."

Saving Strategies
We all have the power to end violence and to heal. Children, parents, caretakers, the power to save the family is within us. Be proactive. Take leadership roles and form Wellness Circles with like-minded youth, youth builders, and youth entrepreneurs and youth freedom fighters. Form vegetarian/vegan groups. Grow organic food and herbs in community gardens, window sill planters and backyard gardens. Form or join a Food Co-op to assure access to quality, affordable, organic, GMO-free foods, and fruits with seeds, as opposed to seedless, devitalized, artificially produced fruits (i.e. seedless watermelons, grapes, oranges). Organize healthy circles in community centers, on your block, in your home, and in your schools. Young people, be proactive, decide to be the solution to bring power and prosperity. Raise your frequency daily with positive productive thoughts. Dwell in the circle of positive, productive people who are about building vibrant, radiant lives.

Brain Power

The most powerful circle is within you and that circle is your brain. The brain, the headquarters of the body, sends messages to the entire anatomy. The condition of the brain is the condition of one's life. It indicates whether one will be healthy or diseased; whether one attracts pain or wellness. As we help our children rejuvenate the brain we gain a "Supa Brain" and therefore a "Supa Life" of Optimal Wellness. As we charge our children's brains with whole organic vegan food, based on the five elements, we will raise the frequency of our children which will move our children out of harm's way into a high frequency protective zone. (Also see: BRAIN FOOD in Paradigm 3.)

Incorporating the 5 Elements

Ether (consciousness): Perform daily meditation and speak positive, affirmation words of power. Drink Ginko and Gota Kola herbal teas, to rejuvenate the brain.

Air: Oxygenate your entire body. Invert your entire body. Lie down in a 45 degree angle for 10 min 2x daily. Perform 20-50 deep inhalations/exhalations, 2x daily.

Fire: Eat and drink blood builders (i.e. cranberry, blueberries and strawberries)

Water: Flush and saturate your cells, brain and nerves with eight glasses of water, daily.

Earth: Rejuvenate the brain. Consume green foods and green juices daily.

Balance Air and Water Elements

De-stress and comfort your child from worry and fear. Give your youth 2-3 Epsom salt baths, weekly. Have them soak in the tub for 20-30 minutes as they drink 16 oz. of warm water and lime juice. While in the tub give your child 16 oz. of water with 50 mg of vitamin B complex. End the bath with a warm shower. Place shower spray over their chest, face and back to promote deep relaxation and inner peace. To further de-stress have your child perform several deep inhalations and full exhalations. Nourishing the brain with natural elements helps to prevent depression, anxiety, bipolar, mood swings mental confusion and memory loss, which can aid in the prevention of suicide in youth. Nourishing the brain aids in one being spiritually attuned, which will help to keep our children out of the low frequency zone of violence. As we caretakers support our children to obtain healthy "Supa Brain" power your child will experience mental clarity and positive productive thoughts. From productive healthy thoughts one creates a healthy outcome. To maintain the "Supa Brain" power, **do not** feed your child sugar which destroys the brain as well as fast foods and junk foods that clog up the brain. Avoid both polyunsaturated fats that congest the brain and heavy metals that deteriorate the brain. Caretakers, in the interest of protecting and fortifying your child's brain, you, also, must strive to live a "Supa Brain" lifestyle.

Open Your Wellness Home
Once you, caretaker, heal yourself, open your wellness home to help your family and others to heal themselves. Use your Nutrition Kitchen Pharmacy for sharing green juice de-stressors, rejuvenation juices and whole food meals. Use your Live In Room for group sharing, exercise and fitness activates, journal writing, and meditation that not only will protect and support your teen but also you, the adult. I recall when my children were very young I started a "Young Sprout Circle", a holistic lifestyle environment for children to grow well for ages 8–12 and a "Clean Teen Circle" for ages 13–16. It consisted of my children, some of their friends and even some of my clients enrolled their children in our Youth Circles. My own children, from ages 9-13, gave classes in vegan food preparation, yoga and meditation to their young peers. The parents observed the youth classes, read information on holistic living and engaged in discussion circles on topics of wellness.

Open your wellness home to parents who suffer from the pain of having lost a child whose life was taken; to help a parent in trouble; to help a child in trouble. Teach them how to shield and heal their family. Build extended support families with activities such as camping in nature, fitness in the park, visits to the movies and museums. All of these activities can be used to stimulate spiritual growth. I would always say to my children, "Don't hang out, be on mission; be on purpose --for those who hang out can get hung." As families unite in wellness we have a greater ability to protect our children, one child, and one family at a time.

A Community of Wellness

At the close of preparing this book, and in the midst of the tragedy that occurred in Ferguson, Missouri*, a holistic miracle occurred. Khepera Kearse is my dear devoted student, an Ambassador of Wellness and an Emerald Green Holistic Practitioner. Khepera introduced my sons and I into a Circle of Wellness in a Peace Week activity with Erica Ford, founder of Life Camp. Peace Week was sponsored by Russell Simmons who presented a special dinner for mothers who had lost their sons to gun violence. For two decades Erica Ford has been a freedom fighter for saving our children and our communities from violence. She approaches violence as a disease from which the community needs to be cured. Her work has reached the office of the Mayor of the City of New York, President Obama's office, as well as the office of The James E. Davis Stop the Violence Foundation, which, among other things, sponsors the "Love Yourself Stop the Violence Walk". With Erica, my sons and I took model circles of women and men through a 21 Day Challenge based on two of my books: **The City of Wellness** and **Heal Thyself.** Twenty-five students from Erica's camp received my 21 Day Detox Kit. The participants learned to how to set up wellness homes and how to be healers in their homes. We the healers: Supa Nova Slom, Erica Ford, Ali Amechi, Khepera Kearse, Tracy Queen, Doctor Bernadette Sheridan, Dare Special Holistic Opps and I formed a Circle of Wellness and brought about a Community Detox. We joined forces to create the Wellness Model for Global Healing and Transformation. And so it is.

Parents of Wellness, It's Time To Rise!

---

* On August 9, 2014.Michael Brown, an 18 year old unarmed Black teenager, was shot and killed by Darren Wilson, a White police officer, in Ferguson, Missouri. The shooting provoked protests in Ferguson, for weeks. On November 24, 2014 the St. Louis County prosecutor announced that a grand jury decided not to indict Mr. Wilson for the death of Mr. Brown. The announcement provoked protests in major cities across the United States.

(TRANSFORMATION)

ADDRESSING AUTISM

> "Autism is a developmental disorder. Because brain development follows a complicated series of delicately timed events beginning early in gestation and continuing through infancy and into early childhood, "environmental insults" may occur at numerous time-points, each with a distinct imprint in terms of the processes affected and the intensity of the impact. Some of those environmental factors may include things like pesticides; flame retardants; ingredients in household products (incl. air fresheners and cookware); compounds used in plastics as well as in fragrances; food contaminants, or by-products of food processing; micronutrients; metals; and medications, especially those that target the central nervous system."
>
> - *Dr. Irva Herz-Picciotto, CHARGE (Childhood Autism Risks from Genetics and the Environment) The CHARGE Study and The MARBLES Study/ UC Davis MIND Institute/ Sacramento, CA 95817*
>
> "A digestive system which does not contain healthy flora (good bacteria) cannot eliminate toxins, and allows bad things to pass into our bloodstream. It also cannot get the most nourishment from our food. Both have come to the same conclusion: that the modern western diet, which has spread around the world, is essentially the root cause of the worldwide spread of autism and that the cure is already here—one just has to eat the correct food; a mostly plant-based diet with an emphasis on fermented foods."
>
> - *Health Expert, Donna Gates and Dr. Natasha Campbell-McBride.*

The following testimony from a mother who dared to heal her son has inspired me to share with caretakers and parents some suggestions on how to rejuvenate a child's brain and nervous system. Your child diagnosed with Autism could very well become your "miracle child."

Testimony from a Mother Who Dared To Heal Her Son

My name is Phyllis. Fifteen years ago I was desperate to help my son, Bill. The diagnosis from several doctors was that he suffered from Autism and Schizophrenia. I was totally opposed to giving him the pills that were always dispensed to our young black boys who had various issues that caused them to be diagnosed as having Autism. I was determined to get my son off the medication and seek an alternative to those pills they prescribed to him.

My neighbor suggested that I take my son to Queen Afua for a consultation. I went to see her with positive expectations that she would be able to give me hope and offer something for my son that wouldn't have so many side effects. When we visited Queen Afua's office my son was in bad shape. He continually hummed, looked straight ahead with a blank expression, heard voices and was non-responsive. During the consultation, Queen gave my son an herbal drink, and gave me suggestions to change his diet and include natural vitamins. Queen Afua was the first person to tell me about the dangers of white sugar and preservatives in processed foods. I made the changes she suggested.

I give Queen Afua the credit for the shape my son is in today. Bill was 15 years old at the time of that first consultation. Today he is 30 years old. He attends Community College and is preparing to retake his GED test. (He is only 4 points from the completion certificate.) Bill has achieved a green belt in Karate and occasionally is the "praise and worship" leader at his place of worship. Next fall he will be attending a four-year college in New Jersey. I believe because of Queens Afua's wisdom and gift for healing, my son went from taking 80 mg. of prescription medication to 10 mg. and is on his way shortly to taking none.

I thank the Creator for putting Queen Afua, a true queen, in our midst, to stress the importance of healing thyself. May the "Most High" continue to bless Queen Afua and her family and her staff.

Sincerely,
Phyllis

(Transformation)

8 Keys To Wellness For the Brain and Nervous System

Caretakers, Parents and Grandparents Circle Your Child in Wellness

These 8 Keys to Wellness are for nourishing your child's brain and nervous system. Applying them daily will absolutely support your child to have a better quality of life. Be consistent for 21 Days to 1 season of wellness in order to witness a breakthrough. Once you experience the improvement in your child, make the 8 Keys to Wellness a part of life for you, your child and your family. The best way to ensure your child's well-being is to secure the caretaker (yourself) in wellness.

1. Serve your child Green Life Nutritional Formula I. Use 1 to 2 Tbs. of Green Life Formula I (contains Vitamin A, B, D, E, K, vegetable calcium and vegetable protein) a day with 4 oz. of fresh organic apple or pear juice or vegetable juice followed by 4 oz. of distilled or alkaline water. (2-3 x per day)

2. Give your child or teenager 25 mg. of Vitamin B complex in powdered form blended with juice or water. (2x per day)

3. Serve fresh green salads with steamed vegetables. Serve whole grains and vegetable protein (beans, peas, lentils, soaked almonds) and sprouts over a bed of fresh leafy greens. (2x per day)

4. Keep brown and white sugar out of your child's diet. Sugar destroys the brain cells and the nervous system. As a healthy sweet alternative, keep a fruit bowl full of your child's favorite fruit in your Nutrition Kitchen Pharmacy.

5. Become a Food Co-op member or form a Co-op to be able to purchase affordable organic, non-GMO foods at reasonable prices. This will support your effort to serve whole foods for a whole body, mind and spirit.

6. Feed your child's brain: Massage your child's back and head gently, in a clockwise direction with cold pressed olive oil to send energy to your child's brain. (Daily for 10 minutes AM & PM), as you pour love into your childs crown.

7. De-stress Your Child: Before massage give your child a warm water salt bath (1lb. Epsom salts) (15-20 minutes, 3x per week)

8. Keep Your Child's Circulation up to Par: Have your child engage in some form of activity such as sports, biking, running, dance, etc., whatever form of movement that your child can enjoy.

LOVE YOUR CHILDREN...

by Judy Baldaccini

Love your children when they are wrong...
It sets an example of tolerance,
in a world of imperfections.
Love your children when they are hurt...
It sets an example of empathy,
the ability to feel another's pain.
Love your children when they are angry...
It sets an example of compassion, to
all living things.
Love your children when you disagree with them...
It sets an example of acceptance, to those
with differences around us.
Love your children when they lose...
It sets an example of triumph, even in
the face of doubt.
Love your children when they have a temper tantrum...
It sets an example of a willingness, to
accept things beyond our control.
Love your children when they are down...
It sets an example that with time,
all things come to pass.
Love your children when they curse...
It sets an example of forgiveness,
allowing goodness to prevail.
Love your children when they have shame...
It sets an example of humility, how to
live a life as a humble individual.
Love your children when they are happy...
It's contagious!

Judy Baldaccini – is a woman who found her voice, walked away from abuse and continues her journey
of healing as a writer, an artist, and a woman – who found her voice ...

(TRANSFORMATION)

UPLIFT OUR ELDERS

Caretakers of elders, I am sharing this page of my life especially with you. Our parents, grandparents, uncles, aunts and/or perhaps, spouse/mate are aging and need additional care and assistance. We daughters, sons, grandchildren, nieces, nephews and/or significant others, must assume the position of caretaker. Often, this awesome responsibility occurs with little or no warning. Caretakers, you can expect to become overwhelmed and stressed. You may even feel helpless or worse, hopeless. I know; I have been there.

How did we get here? We humans are living longer. Factors such as genetics, diet, exercise and wellness care history have an impact on how we live our lives as the aging process manifests itself. Generally, the challenges to longevity occur in the form of chronic dise-eases and/or in the form of acute episodes. We tend to address symptoms of chronic dis-eases such as diabetes, arthritis and high blood pressure with allopathic medicine or holistic techniques or both. Acute episodes including strokes and heart attacks (often by-products of chronic conditions) are usually treated in the emergency room of the hospital.

CARETAKING OPTION ONE:
Following long-term or short-term hospitalization treatment, the next step is usually transfer to a nursing home facility for rehabilitation. Depending both on their health and financial circumstances an elder might experience multiple transfers between the hospital and the nursing home. While your loved one is in these facilities you are no longer primary caretaker. The type and amount of care that is given is no longer in your hands. Additionally, your work schedule and other life obligations will determine how frequently you will be able to visit. With limited family interaction many elderly people feel abandoned, lonely and unloved and give up the will to live.

CARETAKING OPTION TWO:
You might decide to keep the elder at your home or theirs. Either way, in this situation, especially if unprepared, the caretaker quickly becomes overwhelmed,

stressed, fatigued, depressed and angry. Furthermore, as the elder becomes sicker and more dependent, often, the at-home caretaker equally becomes physically and emotionally weakened.

CARETAKING OPTION THREE:
You might opt to receive holistic education in order to circle your elder in wellness and halt the health challenges usually associated with the aging process. To actively pull your elderly family member out of despair, facilitate their healing process and protect yourself as caretaker, I *strongly* recommend that you apply the techniques suggested on the chart at the end of this message. I know; I have been there.

At 90 years old my mother had lucid mental and conversational skills, normal blood pressure and without assistance was able to walk from room to room in her brownstone home, wash clothes, sweep her kitchen floor and prepare her own food. Then, one morning she awoke with pain in her legs and was unable to get out of her bed. Over the next few days she was in excruciating pain and totally dependent for all her needs and care. We took her to the hospital. After she was in the hospital for six weeks we were advised to take her to a nursing home as there was nothing else they could do for her. At the nursing home she fell and was returned to the hospital. Once again, after a short time hospital authorities told us there was not much they could do to help my mother. We brought mother home. My brother informed my son and I that according to the medical statistics we had 30 days to "turn her around" or she would have to be placed back in a nursing home. With that, he wished us, "good luck", turned on his heels and left. Feeling hopeless and distressed, my brother thought, at best, our mother would live the rest of her days –not for long– in a nursing home. He began preparing for mother's funeral.

My sons and daughter and I decided to encircle my mother and her health issues holistically. As a family we prepared herbal tonics and teas and juice therapy, administered healing baths and performed hands-on exercises. During her *twelve week* recovery I also made certain that my mother received a series of healing massages to increase her blood circulation. I was excited about aiding my mother to wellness; more importantly she became more and more hopeful.

(Transformation)

Because I am an energized, holistically aware caretaker and my children were being totally supportive, my mother has recovered from being completely bedridden and barely responsive. We were able to relieve the swelling in her legs and ankles and restore her mind from the intermittent symptoms associated with Alzheimer's disease. Her mental recall has become totally lucid and optimally functional; her high blood pressure is now normal. The doctors, nurses and my brother all were astonished when my mother fully recovered. In *twelve weeks* my mother was able to walk again. She is smiling again while working in my home lab. Without assistance, she is fully able to walk from room to room, wash clothes, sweep her kitchen floor and prepare her own food. On my mother's 90th birthday, in 2013, she gleefully affirmed that she wants to reach the age of 100. In December 2014 my mother celebrated her 91st birthday. I wholeheartedly believe that if she continues to drink her wellness tonics, apply her clay packs, take her soaking baths and perform her exercise schedule, she will reach her goal of living to 100 years in wellness.

Caretakers and care-taking families, seek consultation, co-ordinate your time and support each other. I know for certain that if you encircle your elders in wellness that you will not become a broken, overwhelmed caretaker, but rather with nature's support, you will become an amazing, energized and enthusiastic caretaker. I wish you great fortune as you perform your holistic miracle in a circle of love and wellness. ...I know, Beloveds; I have been there.

Editor's PS: This is a testimonial to the *MANY* caretakers of our elders. Two of them are my youngest sister, Phyllis and my sister-friend, Queen Afua.

Phyllis and our mother, GrandMary live in Florida. In mid 2014, six months after her 90th birthday, GrandMary was diagnosed with "suspicious cells" in her uterus. When the first doctor suggested surgery my sisters and I said, "No." A second doctor, who agreed with the "no surgery" vote, prescribed radiation therapy. He said she was a "strong ninety" and with the entire medical staff was amazed at GrandMary's overall appearance and wellness "for a woman her age." GrandMary and Phyllis were **Magnificent Ones** from Queen Afua's 2009 program. They were thoroughly familiar with holistic living and alternative health care. Except for swimming in pools with chlorine, the doctor supported continuing "alternative" strategies during the seven weeks of radiation therapy. To GrandMary and Phyllis this meant living as **Magnificent Ones,** full throttle. For seven weeks, Phyllis juggled transportation, food preparation and managing her Thai Yoga Studio with getting our mother through the therapy. Suddenly, their mother-daughter circle had new dimensions; new lessons. It was the first time Phyllis had to care for a 90 year-old on radiation therapy; the first time GrandMary *was* a 90 year-old on radiation therapy. They tried to stay positive, radiation side-effects and all. GrandMary continued making her second thousand Origami cranes and her handmade greeting cards. She crocheted purses from the "plarn" she created from plastic bags. It took time for the women to overcome the challenges of fear, frustration and just plain old being exhausted. Their "Health Care Is Self Care" training, the support of wonderful friends, and Skype calls "home" to Brooklyn helped them to survive and excel. Now that the therapy is over, my mother's "clean bill of health" shows the absence of cancer. She is anxious to get back on her tricycle and back into the swimming pool. She and Phyllis are committed to "living green" and continuing to cultivate circles of wellness.

And then there is my sister-friend. Queen Afua wrote the story of the process of uplifting her mother to wellness. But she omitted an heroic and almost unbelievable piece of the story. In 2013, Queen's mother (affectionately called "Grandmother") and my mother, GrandMary, each turned ninety years old two months apart. Grandmother, in a stylish outfit was a beautiful guest at my mother's birthday party, where they were *not* the only **nonagenarians** in the room. I have personally witnessed Grandmother sweeping, cooking, and socializing and we frequently speak on the phone about our mutual love of a luxurious bath. The week before she was hospitalized I saw Grandmother gardening in front of her home. So, imagine my alarm when I called there and was told that Queen and Ali had taken Grandmother to the hospital because she woke up with tremendous pain in her legs and was unable to get out of bed. For the three months that Grandmother was in the hospital and nursing home, Queen Afua's dedicated commitment to her "Health Care Is Self Care" philosophy was put to the test. Her typical day began near dawn, included multiple activities for QAWC, on-site consultations, and teleconference workshops that ended well after 8 PM. Family, friends and staff were in place to assist with all of this, except one last thing. During Grandmother's hospital stay, every night when Queen "finished work" she got on her bike and peddled over two miles each way to the hospital to attend to her mother. When she arrived at the hospital, she secured her bike in the ambulance bay; donned her white jacket (in her backpack, along with tonics, green clay and massage oils) and took the elevator to the floor where her mother was. Thus came about Queen's *circle* of providing holistic care to her mother. Rain or shine Queen made the five-mile round trip to reconnect her mother to a Circle of Wellness. The tonics and clay and massage therapy Queen provided went a long way to setting the foundation for Grandmother's eventual recovery. Queen sees the entire experience as "a miracle." I see Queen as "A Healing Angel on Wheels", circling the community.

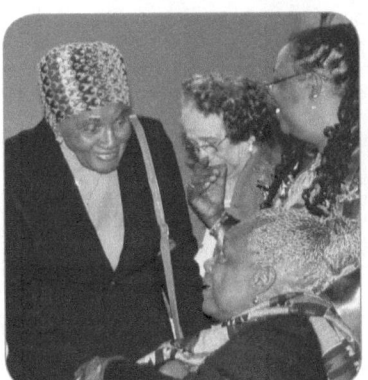 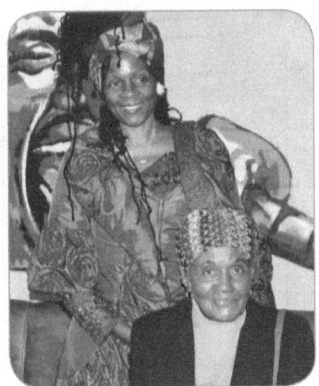

GrandMary's 90th Birthday Party 11/24//13
Left: Grandmother & GrandMary. Right: Queen & Grandmother

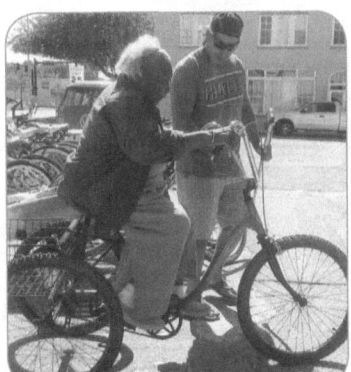 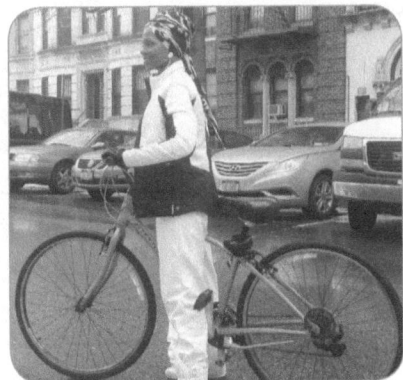

Left: GrandMary on tricycle Birthday 91 Fall/2014. Right: Queen Afua on bicycle Winter/2015.

Checklist for Taking Care of Elders

NOTES: Join other families also caring for elders. Join a Food Co-op to make it easier and more economical to purchase fresh foods. Provide your elders fresh food, especially steamed and juiced turnips to strengthen their back. Wash fruits w/cider vinegar and sea salt. Make sure the elder is drinking water. Use chart below.

Dis-ease(s)	Daily Acts of Wellness	Foods To Avoid
Arteries	Drink Alkaline water. Drink warm water with juice of 2 limes daily	Sugar
Swollen ankles	Foot soaks with Mater Herbal Tonic. Apply clay packs over ankles & feet with gauze overnight. Rinse off in morning shower	Fried foods and meat
Swollen legs & inability to walk	Healing baths or showers (only if elder has help)	Fried foods and meat
Memory and mental challenges that are symptomatic of Alzheimer's / Dementia	Drink the Green Life Nutritional Formula 2–3 times a day to rejuvenate the brain and the entire anatomy	Sugar; white flour products that convert into sugar
High Blood Pressure	Drink Master Herbal Tea	Fried foods, meat and late night eating
Constipation	Take Colon Ease Formula III with lime & warm water Take Herbal Laxative IV	Bread and other white flour starches ie. white rice, white bread etc.
Diabetes	Apply clay packs with Rejuvenation Clay V and gauze over feet and fingers overnight 3x a week, shower next day. Apply clay over eyes with gauze for 2 hours then shower. Perform 2x a week.	Sugar; white flour products that convert into sugar; fried foods
Erectile Dysfunction (Male) Prolapsed Womb (Female)	Daily exercise, i.e., walking	Meat, dairy, fried foods, junk & processed food

(Transformation)

Juice Therapy	Nature's Cure
1 part each: turnip, kale bunch, broccoli bunch	Apply Rejuvenation Green Clay V over affected area overnight for 21 days shower off in the morning
Cucumber, watercreess, parsley	Massage at least 3x a week; Invert legs for 10 minutes 2 x a day (do not invert if person has high blood pressure)
½ turnip juiced in green drink 3x a week	Rejuvenation Green Clay V packs over swollen areas
Add dark green leafy veggies, kale, spinach. Drink 1–2 glasses of water after every glass of juice	Green Life: 1–2 Tbs. in water 2–3 times a day Gota Kola, Ginko
Juice all dark green leafy veggies	3 Tbs. Master Herbal Formula to 3 cups of water; Walking to stimulate blood circulation; Arm swings and leg swings. AVOID INVERSION
Apple juice	Abdominal Massages; Enemas; Be sure to include in diet: Water, Flaxseed, Okra, Fresh Apples & Pears. Puree fruits if eating raw problematic due to dentures
Juice, Bitter Melon, String Beans	Walk begin w/2 steps, then 4, then up to 10 and ultimately around the block. Walk w/ them until they can walk on their own. Burdock, Golden Seal, Master Herbal II –alternate weeks. Inversion exercise if no HBS. Massage abdomen in circular motion/21 circles w/ palm
Green juice 8–16 oz with 1 Tbs Green Life and water	Man's Herbal Formula, Leg Raises, Inversion exercise if no HBS, Leg Swings, Biking (Lie On Back And Do Peddle motion)

Be at peace, your elders nursed you when you were a baby, now it's time to nurse them.
From Queen Afua with Love.

(PARADIGM SHIFT 2)

UNIFICATON

Cultivating Allopathic and Holistic Circles

"Arrange For Me The Way.
May I Renew Myself,
May I Become Strong."

from The Papyrus of Ani

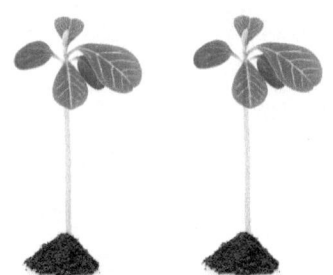

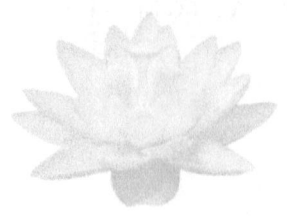

A NEW WAY OF LIFE

We walked in…
Some on canes,
some slowly,
some quicker than others
We walked in
To be shut in
To listen
To learn
We walked in
To get rid of some weight
We walked in
To look better
To feel better
We walked in
To change our lives
We walked in
To change our eating habits
We walked in
To change
We walked in
And walked out
Changed forever with a new lifestyle
and a new way of life.

by Elaine Pinckney
(Magnificent Ones/April 2009)

(UNIFICATION)

IT BEGINS WITH DOCTOR DAVIDSON

Doctor Ronald Davidson, a friend and colleague, a medical doctor, and a holistic physician passed on into the Ancestral realm in June 2006; he was 54 years young. His solid commitment to combining Eastern and Western approaches to health care actually helped to prolong his own life as he battled an aggressive and debilitating illness. The entire community admired his laser sharp mind and his hard work, as well as the bond he had with his patients. In his Brooklyn and Manhattan clinics he had merged allopathic with holistic practices decades before it became fashionable to do so.

He quickly and quietly moved from patient to patient giving them the best of his allopathic and holistic expertise. He took care of us. After writing a prescription for diabetic patients he would insist they begin the exercise portion of their healing right then and there on the stationery bicycle in his clinic. He understood the importance of cultural celebration and artistic expression through music and dance and set up "concerts" performed and attended by his patients. The concerts were healing for his patients and the community at large. Dr. Davidson fully embraced the concept and taught the community to Heal Thyself. The fact that he never said, "No," to any of us resulted in him living his life as a Healing Juggernaut...a Wellness Warrior in the truest sense.

It was Dr. Davidson who opened his doors to me to work in his clinic in the 1970s and 1980s, when I was but a neophyte in the Holistic Health field. I worked with his patients sharing my growing knowledge of holistic approaches to attain wellness for body, mind and spirit. Although he wholeheartedly supported blending allopathic with holistic practices, at the time neither of us was financially prepared to launch the very costly clinical trial needed to prove the validity of East meets West for relief from illness and disease.

For over two decades I searched for the opportunity for the clinical trial to be born. Then I met Dr. Bernadette Sheridan. Dr. Davidson would be pleased.

BOTH OF THEM

This chapter begins with the story of how two healers formed a circle. In 2009 Queen Afua and Dr. Sheridan combined their skills to demonstrate that "Health Care Is Self Care". With over 20 participants and a "Dream Team" of holistic and allopathic assistants, they conducted a three-month project called The Magnificent Ones. The success of the project included medical monitoring (Dr. Sheridan) and holistic guidance (Queen Afua), both at the world-class level. They continue to work together to support those seeking the flagship concept: Heal Thyself.

MEET DR. BERNADETTE SHERIDAN

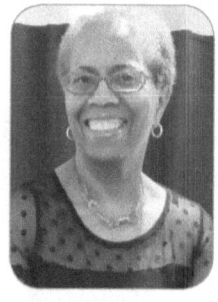

A Board-certified physician practicing family medicine for over 30 years, Dr. Bernadette Sheridan is the founder/director of Grace Family Medical Practice located in Brooklyn, New York. She received her undergraduate degree from Johns Hopkins University and her M.D. degree from the State University of New York at Buffalo. Diverse experiences including service on an Indian reservation and with prison populations helped shape her desire to provide comprehensive Family Practice care.

Balancing career goals, family and self-fulfillment, Dr. Sheridan serves families to experience disease prevention, early detection, disease management and patient empowerment.

A Diplomat of the American Academy of Family Practice, she maintains a leadership position as a physician reducing the gap in health disparities. Dr. Sheridan, who appropriately deserves her many awards and her consistent place on the list of New York's "Top Doctors", is also a member of the Overseas Medical Assistance Team, a group of Doctors and Health Care Professionals who volunteer their time for annual trips to Underserved Areas of the Caribbean and

Africa. Dr. Bernadette Sheridan is a global physician who has become legendary as a passionate wellness advocate to thousands of patients in the United States and around the world.

Meet Queen Afua

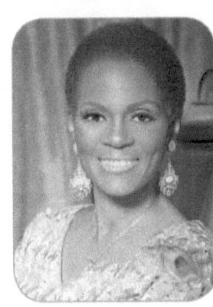

Queen Afua is internationally renowned and certified holistic health practitioner, an author and a devoted wellness advocate. She is also a certified colonic therapist, fasting specialist and a yoga instructor. Based in Brooklyn, New York, Queen Afua has built a wellness empire that includes The Queen Afua Wellness Center (QAWC), The Heal Thyself Green Living product line and The Global Sacred Woman Village.

Nearly 40 years ago Queen Afua opened a small holistic center and wrote some guides for fasting and detoxification. The center grew. The guides became best-sellers including, *Heal Thyself: For Health and Longevity; Sacred Woman: A Guide to Healing the Feminine Body, Mind & Spirit* and *The City Wellness: Restoring Your Health Through the Seven Kitchens of Consciousness*. With texts, consultations, seminars and holistic products that she has created, Queen has assisted thousands to reverse dis-ease challenges and embrace their wellness. World-wide leaders and celebrities have invited her to present her wellness acquisition program in private homes and public venues. She does so – alone and/or with members of the Heal Thyself family; in churches and/or in theaters and through telecommunication. For an hour, a day, a season; for four decades…around the globe!

Queen Afua's detoxification and purification programs have been clinically tested and approved by prestigious doctors. It is not surprising that the joys of her life – dance, nature and her grandchildren – inspire her work and are skillfully and lovingly incorporated into her strategies for wellness.

WE MEET

In 2008 I received a call from Dr. Bernadette Sheridan, founder and director Head Physician of Grace Family Practice. We had in common my client, her patient, who referred us to each other. I answered this long-awaited call and traveled to Grace Family Practice to meet this well sought after physician. Upon arrival I got on and off the elevator and walked right into the arms of Doctor Sheridan, and she into mine. We held onto one another for what felt like a lifetime. It was pure peace, respect, humility and joy flowing to and from Medical Practitioner and Holistic Practitioner. We hugged, we looked at each other, we smiled; in that moment each breathing in the possibilities. After spending four hours of sharing our thoughts and hopes of finding, "someone like you", we knew that we could and would work together for the common good of the people. The impact of our unity would come to symbolize the magnificence of transformation into a new way of wellness acquisition.

Doctor Sheridan wanted to meet because several of her long-time patients were improving. She asked them the classic question, "What are you doing differently?" They would say without fear, "I am on Queen Afua's 21 Day Detox Program." They also let her know that, as my clients I never discouraged them from following their physician's instructions. There was no conflict; the client did not have to choose between their physician and their holistic practitioner. Dr. Sheridan was looking at a holistic practitioner who could work with her, while remaining a master of her craft. She understood that I would not jeopardize her work. I, on the other hand had been searching for years for a physician who could believe in my work to the point of assisting to bring forth a clinical trial to prove that my work, the 21 Day/12 week Detox Program, was a safe, effective and practical way to rejuvenate families holistically.

After our meeting, I volunteered to teach a series 90 minute Holistic Workshops at Dr. Sheridan's clinic. These workshops, based on the Empowerment Wheels of Wellness I had created, covered everything from prevention of arthritis to prevention of diabetes, high blood pressure, fibroids, impotency, and more. (See The 12 Empowerment Wheel Circles in Paradigm Shift 4 in this text). I was invited by Dr. Sheridan to teach her patients and staff at Grace Family Practice. After one year of Wellness Donation, I asked Dr. Sheridan if we could begin a clinical trial. She responded, "I am the scientist, you create the healing program and I will test its effectiveness." So that all the people would have an equal opportunity to be in the trial, regardless of their economic status, Dr. Sheridan and I offered our services pro-bono. Additionally, she recruited Dr. Rita Strickland, RN and four other volunteer nurses and together with members of my staff a Dream Team of volunteers offered their services pro-bono as well. We all took the journey with open hearts and without salaries because we believed in the possibility of offering an alternative program that could become a staple in restoring the underserved and the served, the insured and the uninsured. The test was completed on 21 women and men (2 independent participants) for 12 weeks.

Dr. Sheridan said: "Since our collaboration began, Queen Afua and I have sought ways to incorporate her knowledge and expertise with my practice of medicine. We firmly believe that holistic and allopathic do not have to be natural enemies. The two disciplines can come together in mutual respect and the end product will be wellness for the people. Especially for populations at risk ... from diabetes at amazing rates, with the younger ones joining the ranks faster than the older ones ..., we continue to strive to empower people to help their practitioners heal themselves."

Of course, you know that this is not without its challenges and pitfalls, too numerous to categorize here, but we decided to use this venue to ask the question: Is it Possible?

HEALTH REPORT CARD

The following are statistics regarding challenges to health, particularly to People of Color in the US and the Caribbean.

Heart Disease
African American men are 30% more likely to die from heart disease. African Americans are 1.5 times as likely to have high blood pressure.

Cancer
African American men are 1.4 times as likely to have new cases of lung and prostate cancer and 2.4 times as likely to die from prostate cancer. African American women are 10% less likely to have been diagnosed with breast cancer; however, they are 36% more likely to die from breast cancer.

Stroke
African American adults are 30% more likely to have a stroke. African American males are 50% more likely to die from a stroke.

Diabetes
African Americans were 2.1 times more likely to have been diagnosed with diabetes and are 2.1 times more likely to die from diabetes.

HIV/AIDS
African Americans make up only 13% of the population, but they accounted for over 50% of all U.S. HIV/AIDS cases in 2004.

Overweight and Obesity
African American men and women make up 69.3% of the overweight or obese population in the United States.

(UNIFICATION)

About 70% of children in the United States will contract **Respiratory Syncytial Virus** (RSV) by the time they are one year old and nearly all children will have had it before they are two. For most, it's no worse than a common cold, but for babies with high risk factors, RSV can lead to a serious lung infection, and is the leading cause of pneumonia and bronchitis in infants.

> **Hepatitis A & E**
> Both are water-borne viruses.
>
> **Hepatitis B**
> Is blood-borne and communicable. Of the 2 billion infected people, more than 350 million have chronic (lifelong) infections.

Around 3.2 million deaths every year are attributable to complications of **diabetes;** six deaths every minute. WHO estimates the number of people with diabetes, worldwide, in 2000 was 171 million and is likely to increase to at least 366 million by 2030.

WHO reports that the disease burden will increase to 60% by the year 2020; **heart disease, stroke, depression, cancer** will be the largest contributors.

The people cry out for liberation of the body, mind and soul. By forming Circles of Wellness we feed the people hope; we promise deliverance. There can be wholeness. We can change the statistics on our **Health Report Card** by forming Circles of Wellness.

(CIRCLES OF WELLNESS)

THE CO$T OF NOT KNOWING

See the "price tags" below for six surgical procedures regularly performed on women. Some patients argue that these expenses do not come out of their pockets because they have adequate insurance coverage. But what about the price the human body pays during and after a surgical procedure? Many medical doctors agree that the better the body is prepared prior to surgery, the more favorable the outcomes and more rapid and complete the recovery. Ultimately, prevention of surgery would be the most cost effective to both the pocketbook and the human body. With or without surgery a patient may want to consider the benefits of preparing and repairing the body, mind and spirit with holistic wellness tools and strategies. Remember: "Health Care Is Self Care."

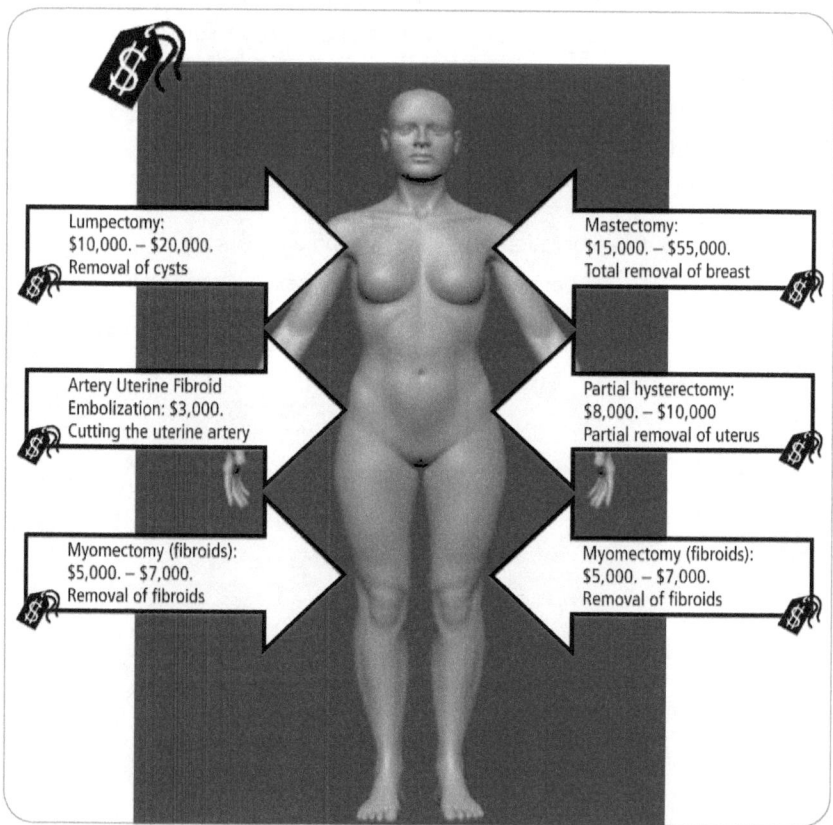

Lumpectomy:
$10,000. – $20,000.
Removal of cysts

Mastectomy:
$15,000. – $55,000.
Total removal of breast

Artery Uterine Fibroid Embolization: $3,000.
Cutting the uterine artery

Partial hysterectomy:
$8,000. – $10,000
Partial removal of uterus

Myomectomy (fibroids):
$5,000. – $7,000.
Removal of fibroids

Myomectomy (fibroids):
$5,000. – $7,000.
Removal of fibroids

(UNIFICATION)

Is It Possible?

Allopathic **Bernadette Sheridan** (Medical Doctor)	Holistic **Queen Afua** (Holistic Practitioner)
Diabetes, Obesity, Depression, High Blood Pressure, Hay Fever… Is it possible that Holistic methods can postpone or improve outcome? **Is it possible?**	People are afraid… Must they choose between Allopathic and Holistic? Can we unite to help families to heal and lead better lives? **Is it possible?**
She has fibroids and they keep coming back. She's asking for alternatives to medications and/or surgery. Is there anything else I can offer her? **Is it possible?**	Women don't believe they can heal with nature. **Is it possible?**
He has prostate challenges and is concerned about cancer and impotency. He's very concerned about having to have surgery and take medications for the rest of his life. **Is it possible?**	Men rarely consider they can heal with nature. **Is it possible?**
Will my colleagues in the Medical Community label me a quack for recommending herbs, clay, and food as medicine? Will I lose my credibility and my reputation that I've worked so hard to establish? **Is it possible?**	Will the Holistic Community label me a traitor if I attempt to merge the Holistic with the Allopathic? Will I lose my credibility and my reputation in the Holistic Community? **Is it possible?**

Will my patients react negatively if I try to tell them how to help heal themselves with foods and natural methods in addition to conventional methods? **Is it possible?**	Will I lose my clients and students if I recommend that they get the support of a medical doctor in addition to my holistic recommendations? **Is it possible?**
Over 30 years of Practicing Medicine. Can we work together? **YES, IT IS POSSIBLE!**	Over 30 years of Holistic Wellness Work. Can we work together? **YES, IT IS POSSIBLE!**

YES, WE CAN UNITE !

YES, IT IS POSSIBLE !

Yes, it is possible, because...

We are on a common path

With a common goal

Not Versus... Side by Side!

"IS IT POSSIBLE?": The performance piece modeled on the real-life experience of Queen Afua and Dr. Sheridan. It was performed by them in **An Evening of Theater That Heals,** a program of vignettes, music and dance. The program was presented on May 6, 2011 at the Producers' Club Theater in Manhattan, NYC, to a gathering of scientists, artists, and healers. The focus of the evening was to create bridges between the medical community and alternative practitioners and to gain the support to create health and educational programs to better serve the needs of the community. Additionally, Dr. Josephine English,* iconic physician and role-model was honored with special tribute. Others in performance: Lady Prema, Mother Sage Sia, Marilyn Worrell, Gerianne Scott, Johanna Figueroa, Empress Thandi, Kuji Lezama-Banks and Katriel-Metaphysical Music Medicine Man. Event supporters included: Safiya Bandele, Dir/Prof Center for Women's Dev MEC; Diana Pharr, Consulting; Dr. Bernadette Sheridan, MD/Founder; Gerianne Scott, Educator/Artist; Marilyn Worrell, Educator/Artist; Leslie & Jason, Wellness Advocates

* Dr. English was the first African American OB-GYN in New York.

(UNIFICATION)

The Proposal And Follow-Up Report

(Excerpts)

Health Care is Self-Care

The Heal Thyself Holistic First Aid Proposal

For Vibrant Communities And Cities Of Wellness In The United States And For Global Cities Of Wellness

By Queen Afua

Sponsored by
Dr. Bernadette Sheridan

… (CIRCLES OF WELLNESS) …

THE HEALTH CRISIS

Our Life & Times

Nearly 50 million Americans have no health insurance. At least 25 million are underinsured. In addition, galloping healthcare costs threaten millions of families with bankruptcy and the risk of losing their homes.

The Need for Heal Thyself Holistic First Aid

The United States health care system is in an all encompassing crisis and is in need of an immediate remedy. Lack of vision is causing ongoing health tragedies in the lives of United States citizens. According to the May 2007 Journal of 119 SEIU, the nation's health care cost this year will top $2.2 trillion. The U. S. healthcare system is the most expensive by virtually every indication and the health of U.S. adults and children trails far behind other industrialized nations.

Twenty percent of the institutions in the League of Voluntary Hospitals are in bankruptcy.

> *"The Patients we serve will have to be absorbed by the existing hospitals of many of our sick, lame and disabled simply have nowhere else to go."*
> — DELEGATE WILLIAM PIGFORD,
> A CLERICAL SPECIALIST AT PRINCE GEORGE'S HOSPITAL

Disease is on the rise... A Doctor Cries Out

What are you willing to change in order to heal your body, mind and spirit?

Are you concerned about the side effects of medication?

Do you want to avoid unnecessary surgery?

(UNIFICATION)

Do you want to lower your blood pressure and/or prevent diabetes?

Do you want to shrink your fibroid tumors?

Would you like to be in control of your weight?

Do you need to resolve an emotional issue?

Do you want better health?

It is time to Heal Thyself.

It is time to come into Circles of Wellness.

— Dr. Bernadette Sheridan, MD

Sign of the Times / The Remedy

The sign of the times is change. The election of an African American to the office of president of the United States is a sign of the times. President-elect Barack Obama, the embodiment of national and global political change, predicts changes in the economy, taxes, employment, education, race relations and last, but not least, health concerns. The Call: On November 5th, 2008, while on CNN, he stated how he wanted to focus on wellness, not medicating. On October 15th, 2008 and throughout the election campaign and debates, then Senator Obama proposed,

> "...in order to save the health of the people and the health of the economy in the United States, we need to consider progressive changes including dis-ease prevention programs offered by community health-care providers..."

I heard the call. For decades, I have been preparing for a time such as this.

— Queen Afua

The Statistics – We Shall Over Come

Ending the Health Disparity in the Most Challenged People: Statistics Say It's Time for Health Reform

African Americans were 2.1 times more likely to have been diagnosed with diabetes and are 2.1 times more likely to die from diabetes. African American men are 30% more likely to die from heart disease; 1.4 times as likely to have new cases of lung and prostate cancer and 2.4 times as likely to die from prostate cancer. African American women are 10% less likely to have been diagnosed with breast cancer; however, they are 36% more likely to die from a stroke. African American men and women make up 69.3% of the overweight or obese population in the U.S.

The General Population / Aiding the Un-Insured and Under-Insured

Around 3.2 million deaths every year are attributable to complications of diabetes – that's six deaths every minute. WHO estimated the number of people with diabetes worldwide in 2000 was 171 million and is likely to increase to at least 366 million by 2030.

WHO further reports that disease will increase to 60% by the year 2020 and heart disease, stroke, depression and cancer will be the largest contributors.

About 70% of children in the United States will contract Respiratory Syncytial Virus (RSV) by the time they are one year old and nearly all children will have had it before they are two. For most, it's no worse than a common cold, but for babies with high risk factors, RSV can lead to a serious lung infection, and is the leading cause of pneumonia and bronchitis in infants.

Hepatitis A & E are water-borne viruses. Hepatitis B is blood-borne and communicable. Of the two billion infected people in America, more than 350 million have chronic, lifelong infections.

The Vision – The Way Out

Project Goals

Provide affordable, quality health care. **Teach and administer** (w) holistic lifestyle practices. **Integrate, Health Care Is Self Care** Heal Thyself Natural Living methods within patients' existing medical care. **Medically measure** the effects of the program on wellness improvement. **Establish** an ongoing model for proactive access to wellness of body, mind and spirit and prevention of disease. **Help to end health disparities** in the Global African Community and communities at large.

Additional Goals:

- **To prove** scientifically the effectiveness of holistic lifestyle methods in treating and preventing disease.
- **To lower** the risk of diabetes and other debulitating dis-eases through Holistic Lifestyle education
- **To integrate** allopathic medicine with natural / (w)holistic developed by the Heal Thyself Natural Living Program and establish this practice as a global model of wellness for prevention of disease.

Project Objectives

The core of the program and the project used to measure the program's effectiveness is to:

Correct toxic eating habits and adopt natural living lifestyle for optimal wellness.

Address wellness challenges such as, eczema, prostate imbalance, heart disease, anxiety, fatigue and malnutrition (many of us are malnourished!)

Focus on colon wellness as a means to reduce risk and/or progression of disease throughout the body. Include (w)holistic approaches to exercise, hydrotherapy work, rest and self-reflective inventory.

Wellness Objectives
- To improve eating habits from a toxic food to a whole food diet thus enhancing radiant vibrant health and vitality
- Holistically lower the risk of diabetes
- To lower and normalize blood pressure
- To assist overweight participants with easy weight loss techniques
- To clear up skin conditions and enhance vibrant skin
- To shrink fibroid tumors and reduce the risk of hysterectomy
- To reduce arthritic pain
- To reduce the progression of diabetes and restore balance to glucose and insulin levels
- To reduce the number of asthma attacks and other related respiratory diseases
- To reduce the risk of colon cancer and related diseases to the colon and to promote colon wellness through holistic lifestyle education

History-Making Wellness Project: Unifying Allopathic & Holistic

YES WE CAN! Shift from Disease to Wellness
The City of Wellness
Presents

"Health Care is Self Care"
12 Week Disease Prevention & Optimal Wellness Program

Supervised by:
Queen Afua, (W)holistic Practitioner
& Dr. Bernadette Sheridan, M.D., F.A.A.F.P.

Medical Care	(W)holistic Wellness Care
Clinical Analysis of 21 Day / 2 Week Program	Holistic Workshops & Consultations
Supervised by Dr. Sheridan	Supervised by Queen Afua
• Medical Examinations • Ongoing Weigh-Ins • Ongoing blood pressure checks	• Wellness Consultations • Nutrition Kitchen Workshops • Holistic Empowerment Workshops • Fitness Classes

Project Location
The clinical trial was located in Brooklyn, NY
at Grace Family Practice

The Research / The Bridge – Allopathic vs. Holistic

Integrative Method for Reaching Our Wellness Goals

Queen Afua's Heal Thyself (W)holistic Disease Prevention & Optimal Wellness Program will be implemented for research over a 12-week period. Dr. Sheridan will supervise and monitor the medical aspects of the project. The project will be recorded. The integration of Queen Afua's (w)holistic wellness program and Dr. Sheridan's scientific analysis will be history-making and in the spirit of President-elect Obama's call for progressive disease-prevention health-care.

We will be making a giant step toward creating a model for promoting affordable and (w)holistic medical health-care in the United States. Eventually, we can promote affordable, quality wellness in places (here and abroad) where the mortality rate is high and the wellness frequency is low.

The Heal Thyself Holistic 1st Aid Program

...After four decades of Wellness Activism, Queen Afua has developed the Heal Thyself, Health Care is Self-Care Holistic First-Aid Program. This 21-day/12 week training is a Global Wellness model to help end the health disparity of among African Americans, to care for the un-insured and those on a quest to prevent reoccurring surgical procedures and to holistically aid those who, as President Barack Obama has stated, are "over medicated."

(W)holistic Health Reform on the Rise – City to City Global Wellness

Queen Afua's Heal Thyself Lifestyle Wellness Program has touched thousands around the globe. For decades people have learned to use Heal Thyself methods to gain wellness. **To make an impact on health reform by interjecting a (w)holistic health policy into the fabric of health care, there must be scientific evidence.** In a 12-week research project, Dr. Bernadette Sheridan will record and analyze the scientific evidence to validate the efficiency of Queen Afua's holistic lifestyle program.

...

(UNIFICATION)

Health Care Is Self Care

Did you know that for every dis-ease there are herbs, whole foods and live juices in Nature's Pharmacy that can assist in restoring wholeness to the body, mind and spirit?

Through Queen Afua's Heal Thyself Holistic 1st Aid Program:
- **Gain** optimal wellness and establish health goals in a step-by-step, one-on-one private wellness consultation with Queen Afua and from other trained Emerald Green Holistic Wellness Practitioners.
- **Learn** valuable principles on how to release dis-ease from your life with weekly workshops and wellness books.
- **Receive** 12 wellness workshops and gain knowledge on how to prevent: stress, obesity, diabetes, high blood pressure, asthma, eczema, arthritis, fibroid tumors, prostate imbalance, STDs, heart conditions, immune system deficiencies and other health challenges.
- **Empower** your life and family and become charged in wellness as you form CIrcles of Wellness in your home with your family.

Case Project: The Sign of the Times is Change

[From: The City of Wellness Newsletter/December 2008]: The election of an African American to the office of president of the United States is a sign of the times. The sign of the times is change.

The Call: President Barak Obama calls for health care that focuses on wellness, not drugs and surgery. He supports progressive changes to save the health of both the citizens and the economy in the United States.

The Response: Dr. Bernadette Sheridan and Queen Afua formed an allopathic and (w)holistic partnership to enhance wellness, particularly in communities where poor health and funds for wellness are severally challenged. Collectively they have provided over 50 years of health-care, nationally and internationally.

As allies they heed President Obama's urgent call for informed and proactive health care.

History-Making Wellness Project/ Pro Bono Factor

January, 2009. Dr. Sheridan and Queen Afua **launched** The *Magnificent Ones* Wellness Project (based on the Health Care Is Self Care system), **a twelve week project** to chart the progress of participants who would be proactive in their health care. Queen Afua believes, "Yes, We Can shift from disease to optimal wellness!" Dr. Sheridan, who coordinated the allopathic measurement portion of the project predicated that if her patients could, "... eliminate even *half* of the medications they are taking they will have reached a milestone toward optimal health."

Participants in the *Magnificent Ones* project received exemplary services from Queen Afua and Dr. Sheridan, as well as from teams of volunteers. Participants purchased (w)holistic products requisite to the program, however, program instructions as well as, allopathic examinations were *pro bono*. **The pro bono factor establishes the project both unique and history-making.**

Some Project Goals

Provide affordable, quality health care. **Teach and administer** (w)holistic lifestyle practices. Integrate Heal Thyself Natural Living and products with their existing medical care. **Medically measure** the effects of the program on wellness improvement. **Establish** an ongoing model for proactive access to wellness of body, mind and spirit and prevention of disease. **Help to end** health disparities in the Global African Community which will be a model for Global Wellness.

Some Project Objectives

The core of the program and the project used to measure the program's effectiveness **is to: Correct toxic eating habits** and adopt natural living habits for optimal wellness. **Address challenges** to wellness including, but not limited to: overweight, high blood pressure, fibroid tumors, arthritis, diabetes, asthma, eczema, prostate imbalance, heart disease, anxiety, fatigue and malnutrition (many of us are malnourished!) **Focus** on **colon wellness** as a means to reduce risk and/or progression of disease throughout the body. Include (w)holistic approaches to **exercise, work, rest** and **reflection.**

Magnificent Ones

Twenty-seven people began the *Magnificent Ones* project for wellness. Twelve weeks later nineteen people in the group and two people independently completed the study. The twenty–one people listed in the final report will henceforth be known as the original *Magnificent Ones 2009.* **They represent the changes; the signs of** *these* **times.**

The Journey of a Wellness Circle

Who Are The Magnificent Ones? The Magnificent Ones is the name given to the wellness circle consisting of the final 21 participants who completed the 12 week wellness project created by Dr. Bernadette Sheridan (Allopathic MD) and Queen Afua (Holistic Practitioner).

The Purpose: To scientifically measure the impact of Queen Afua's Detoxification and Purification/Natural Living Lifestyle on weight, diabetes, high blood pressure, asthma, cholesterol challenges and other wellness-related issues over a season (84 days). **It was planned** to study 50 people.

- Dr. Bernadette Sheridan and a volunteer team monitored the progress of participants as they followed Queen Afua's 84 Day (one season) program of Detoxification and Rejuvenation.
- **Attendance** was strictly taken.
- We began January 4, 2009 and officially ended 12 weeks later on April 8, 2009.
- We met in Dr. Sheridan's Family Clinic every other Wed. and the alternate Wed. we "met" on a group conference call led by Queen Afua for an hour. She spoke on one of the health concerns, such as diabetes, exercise and rest; hydrotherapy and so forth.

When we went to the Grace Family clinic:

- We jogged and did cardiovascular exercises on several re-bounders. A presentation was given by Dr. Sheridan and/or one of the nurses on the

(CIRCLES OF WELLNESS)

Dream Team about high blood pressure, heart disease and other health challenges. Then we had a lecture from Queen Afua. Chef Ali Torain prepared organic and vegan meals.

- Gerianne Scott taught and guided the participants with journaling exercises.
- Measurement of weight, blood pressure and glucose levels taken by Dr. Sheridan's staff.
- Records were kept and are available.
- A Completion-Graduation ceremony took place on April 26, 2009, the week after Easter

Some Results:
- **Under Doctor's Care** 2 or 3 people were allowed to come off of high blood pressure and diabetes meds. 2 of these were not Dr. Sheridan's patients so their doctors had to approve....AND THEY DID! Several were able to reduce required amount of meds.
- Most of the 19 plus, a few of the nurses and dream team also had desired weight loss.
- There were 19 from Brooklyn (3 of the Brooklynites actually traveled in from PA)
- There were 2 independents (outside of NY)
- There were 4 men; all made it to the end; but only 2 came to graduation.
- There were 15 women in the NY/PA crew and the 2 independents
- My family had the oldest and youngest participants (at the time mom, 85; nephew, 30)
- We, the Scotts, were also the largest family group Mom, sister, her hubby and her son (my nephew).

I wasn't in the 21 count at graduation (officially I was on the Dream Team of assistants, not a Magnificent Ones participant). However, my numbers were recorded, as were those of many members of the Dream Team

Submitted Summer 2009 by Gerianne Scott (Dream Team Administrator)
(Presented In my dual role as project administrator and member of the Scott family –four family members who were participants in the 2009 Magnificent Ones Project)

(UNIFICATION)

HEAL THYSELF / HEALTH CARE IS SELF CARE LIFESTYLE TRAINING

Health Care Is Self Care Wellness action Plan for Wellness		Holistic Health Care Reform Program	
The Problem	**The Solution**	**The Method for Wellness**	**Benefits**
Millions of "low income people" in America are underinsured	Health Care Is Self Care Programming as a Healthy Lifestyle	Seasonal 50–100% 21 Day 4 Modular Lifestyle Empowerment Detox & Rejuvenation Program Self Help / Teleconference / Hands-On	Equal Health Care for the Insured & Uninsured
No choice policy / only recognizes & honors allopathic medical treatment	Freedom of choice through Holistic lifestyle training & Allopathic Awareness	Holistic 1st Aid Care for Personal & Family Care Self Help Training manuals & textbooks	Freedom of Choice
Insured with Overmedicated Unnecessary Surgical Procedure	Lifestyle Wellness Program	Food As Medicine The 5 Elements for Disease Prevention	Surgical & Drug Prevention Healthy Body, Mind & Spirit

Health Care Is Self Care Wellness action Plan for Wellness (cont.)		Holistic Health Care Reform Program (cont.)	
The Problem	**The Solution**	**The Method for Wellness**	**Benefits**
American Obesity Epidemic Empty Calories = Malnourishment	Value in the Food Raise the Quality & Frequency of Health	4 Food Groups vs. The 8 Pyramids of Wellness; Consume Nutritionally Rich Food & The Body Will Need Less Portions	Obesity Prevention: Obesity-Free Mentally, Emotionally & Physically Balanced State of Being Heal Thyself Holistically in the City of Wellness
Health Care Economic Hardship or the People & the Economy	Offer Insurance for patients who choose the Heal Thyself method of Natural Living	Form Circles of Wellness Based on Each One Teach One	Affordable Health Care
Health Disparity within the African Communities Overall / Other Communities	Food as medicine 4 Modular Scientific Holistic Research	Prepare Whole Foods from the 7 Kitchens of Consciousness Flexitarian, Vegetarian, Vegan, Live Food Juice Therapy	Less Health disparity in health challenged communities Closing the Health Disparities Gap in Communities of Color
Wide Spread of Infectious Dis-ease	Organic Food Co-Op Backyard Community Lot Farming; Consumption of whole vegetarian / vegan food	12 Circle Guide to Wellness	Immune Booster

Health Care Is Self Care Wellness action Plan for Wellness (cont.)		Holistic Health Care Reform Program (cont.)	
The Problem	The Solution	The Method for Wellness	Benefits
Stress as a Global Disease Violence Prevention	Holistic Fitness at Work Force to Home De-Stress	Holistic Fitness / Nutrition Kitchen / Visual Aids / DVDs & Wellness Charts	De-stress Peaceful Self in the World and at Home
Over Medicated Increase of Drugs	Create Circles of Wellness to Spread Wellness Globally for Holistic, Vibrant Families Globally	Holistic 1st Aid Training to empower families	Drug & Surgical Prevention Avoidance of Side Effects

WEIGHT LOSS TESTIMONIAL

Before I begin my testimony I must pay homage to my sister, Sacred Women Helen AST Walker for introducing me and my family to health and wellness. She consistently shared her knowledge of detoxing and cleansing our systems and urged us to change our eating habits. I want to thank her from the bottom of my heart.

Prior to entering the City of Wellness... I was... a total wreck. Because of life's circumstances, I had allowed my health and well-being to get out of control. I was filled with so many emotions – depressed all the time and lonely. These feelings manifested themselves in other ways, mainly eating. I began eating out of control, eating all times of the night, eating bad food combinations, etc. My friend once said I was the chunkiest vegetarian he has ever known. The next thing I knew the weight started coming on, and no matter what I tried the situation was getting worse. As the weight gain and the unhealthy eating progressed, so did the depression, low self esteem and pain in my leg and lower back. Also, I began getting sick with uncontrollable coughs, constant colds...

blood pressure out of control. I was taking more and more pain killers and relying heavily on a cane.

I was open and ready for a change in my life. I was emotionally drained, I was tired of being overweight, tired of being sick, tired, of not thinking straight, tired of making the wrong decisions, just plain tired of the way my life was heading. My first visit with Dr. Sheridan was a definite reality check, I weighed in at 190 pounds, my BMI was 43.7% and my blood pressure was 174/100. After this reality check I was determined to do whatever it took to gain control of my health and well being. I plan on going forward, not backward with my life.

Mildred Moore
Magnificent Ones/April 2009

Restoring My Health Testimonial

During the month of December, I had to make a decision about my health, but saw no way out being a prisoner of late night eating and sleep deprivation. I attended a meeting about a wellness program that would help me to heal, cure and above all, live differently. I so badly needed this teaching and support to the wellness that would save and extend my life.

January 4, 2009 Queen Afua and her team began teaching about setting up our kitchen to get ready for the wellness journey. I was excited to be one of the Magnificent Ones.

Wednesday January 7, 2009 was our first day of receiving our product and instruction the cleansing and eating correctly would start the next morning.

January 8, 2009 my day started at 6:00 AM with the colon cleanser. (I had to get used to the taste…I did.) Time management was my biggest problem; I was determined to master that with regards to eating better. I remained on task the first week –the hardest week– but felt better. Eight days into my wellness I was

Unification

able to stop taking one of my diabetes medications and within two weeks I lost 12 pounds. I was thrilled and motivated to raise the bar to achieving my goal. Many things changed for me during those weeks with the support from Doctor Sheridan, Queen Afua and the Dream Team. I was able to stop taking my other diabetes medication. Shed tears of joy each week that I lost more weight and felt myself walking lighter, my skin was looking better, my clothes were fitting loosely, and I added more exercise to my wellness. The first time I was able to cross my legs comfortably at the knees I smiled and laughed out loud because it has been several years since I was able to sit comfortably with less pain.

Two weeks ago I was able to wear pants that I had hidden in my closet for a few years. The best gifts are from my friends and family about the way I looked. My children said that I walked faster and climbed the stairs faster. When I my daughter, Courtney asked about my weight loss each week, her question filled my heart with joy.

The cooking classes offered the opportunities to learn more about creating dishes that I would not have eaten before this journey. I learned to juice vegetables. I was thrilled to learn how to prepare dishes that were green, healthy and tasty. I learned to eat less meat and how to prepare raw meals using tofu, soy, proteins and the right seasoning to enhance flavors. I added Green Life to my diet and stopped eating beef, pork, chicken, seafood, eggs, cheese and sugar. Most mornings the Green Life liquid breakfast and Master Herbal tea kept me filled until lunch time. I was on my journey to becoming a vegan.

This season is coming to a close and I am pleased and honored to say that I have lost 33 pounds and I'm looking forward to the final week. I plan to continue on this path. My life is much calmer, no more late night eating, and my sleeping has gotten better. I have told friends, strangers, and family about Queen Afua's Wellness program that changed my thinking, eating and getting well. My diabetes is under control and Dr. Sheridan is pleased with the progress I have made. The soul sweat was an eye opener and I look to experiencing this hydrotherapy cleansing treatment again. Each season I will continue this lifestyle I have chosen to live.

(CIRCLES OF WELLNESS)

Thank you very much, Queen Afua for your vision and teaching. Above all to Bernadette my mentor, sister, friend, and doctor I say, "I love you and thank you for extending the hand that has changed my life for the better.

Elaine I. Pinckney
Magnificent Ones/April 2009

FIVE YEARS LATER...
Email –March, 2014

Greetings Beloved Magnificent Ones,

Can you believe it has been 5 years? I would like to extend a special invitation to you to join me, Queen Afua and

Dr. Bernadette Sheridan of the Grace Family Practice on Sunday, April 27th from 2PM to 6PM for 1 Day Detox to get ready for Spring Cleaning. Please try to join us in reunion and take the opportunity to meet and greet new members of the Wellness Family. Come as you are...bring a friend.

In wellness,
Queen Afua

(UNIFICATION)

Testimonial from Florida

April, 2014

Dear Queen Afua and Dr. Sheridan,

Tell the Magnificent Ones and Wellness Family that GrandMary and I said hello, and we are toasting them with Green Life and Master Herbal Tea. Here's to your optimal health, and well being. CHEERS! We can't believe it's been 5 years either. We are now living in Florida… loving the weather. We are still on our wellness journeys, me at age 58 and Mom at age 90. Yes, we have our challenges from time to time, but still forge on…

We feel blessed to have been given the opportunity to heal ourselves with the guidance of Heal Thyself, and The City of Wellness. It is an ongoing journey that includes fresh air, walking more often, and exercising at the fitness center. We do Yoga, aqua-robics, swimming, exercise classes, and even Zumba, Wepa! (Yipee!)

GrandMary has gone "over the top" in the crafts department, and after I graduated from the Magnificent One Project I studied and have become a Thai Massage Practitioner. We opened a Yoga Studio for Thai Yoga Massage and Kundalini Yoga Classes. The various arts and crafts by GrandMary and other family and friends are displayed and sold at the studio. So, if you are ever in the area stop by and visit us. We miss you and wish we could join the reunion today.

We are there in spirit! Blessings to All.

With Loving kindness,

Phyllis and GrandMary
Magnificent Ones /2009

Living Testimonial

April 27th, 2014

On that day, ten members of the Magnificent Ones and the Dream Team, were present at the Magnificent Ones Reunion. Also present were about twenty community members who responded to the invitation for a One Day Detox and Rejuvenate for wellness. Six women were sitting together. When it was time for group sharing, a young woman, 28 years old, stood up with tears in her eyes and said, "I was just diagnosed with breast cancer and I'm so afraid." Suddenly, one of the elder women stood up to comfort and console the younger woman and she said, "All of us had breast cancer, so we understand what you are going through. We have a breast cancer empowerment circle that you can come into. We'll help you."

The elder woman hugged the younger woman and the heart circle was secured.

This was a moment, I thought to myself. If we can catch these women and educate them on breast cancer prevention and form circles and teach them about the Breast Cancer Prevention Wellness Wheel in this text, we can save our breasts as a global circle of women. I also thought, what a beautiful elder to have embraced the younger woman in such a way, to let her know she's not alone. it was clear to me that in order to unify the allopathic and holistic medicine, Circles of Wellness must continue in order to bridge the gap and lead us all into holistic, healthy, living.

(UNIFICATION)

Excerpts from:

The Magnificent Ones Commencement Exercise Address
(with clinical report statements)

from Dr. Bernadette Sheridan

Friends, distinguished guests, Queen Afua & the Dream Team staff, Magnificent Ones Class of 2009...

Namaste. First, let me commence by thanking the Creator who saw fit to bring us together in this special way and provide us with the tools, to quote Queen Afua, *to Heal Ourselves*. I am so pleased and honored to be here today. This is more than just a happy occasion... These individuals made a commitment to invest in their own personal health using principles of wellness over a 12-week period. The results, while very encouraging, by no means reflect the impact that has been generated on a personal level. It has been my assignment, as the Medical Doctor, to evaluate the program for its scientific soundness, and monitor changes of improvement along the way. ...I can honestly say that each and every person that pushed off from the starting line has been touched as they passed the finish line. Some have been miraculously transformed. Some have been transformed on intangible levels that cannot be measured by the parameters of the study... I can safely say that ALL the characters, students, instructors, support staff, family members, including the "Lead Investigators" Queen Afua and myself, have been affected by this 12 week journey.

This project, like any other thing in life began with a thought in someone's mind. In the case of the *Magnificent Ones*, it was born out of the concern and frustration of two practitioners – one holistic, one allopathic. For the (quarter of a century plus) that I have practiced in Brooklyn, I have watched as technology advanced and statistics dismally worsened. My patient base for the most part is located in Brownsville – East New York, Brooklyn, and largely African-American / Caribbean / Hispanic; I observed how the latest new pharmaceutical advances or procedures didn't seem to be stemming the tide of disease in this location much at all. Whatever the national statistics were for mortality from hypertension, diabetes, or heart disease was exponentially elevated in Brooklyn and astronomically elevated in the population I treated. The dreaded specter of HIV arrived full-blown in Brooklyn in the 80s, further added to the mortality statistics. The books, medical seminars and lectures taught me to "preach a healthy lifestyle" but nowhere in medical school had I been taught exactly *how* to do it. Even when one made a valiant attempt to eat fresher food, one could not escape that which was radiated, sprayed with pesticides, injected with hormones, gassed with toxic chemicals, or genetically engineered. Most of the medical community frowned at the validity of holistic medicine, and frankly, a lot of what my patients shared with me (from internet and other sources) had no value whatsoever, and in some cases was harmful.

The 21st Century did little to stem the tide. Diabetes had now claimed the children. I was seeing newer and younger diabetics, hypertension was showing up in stressed-out teenagers and in parents who struggled to hold it down for their families. Prostate cancer was arriving at age 45 instead of 60 and 70. Colon cancer was appearing without warning, and breast cancer never took a holiday. Things that I only read in textbooks or saw once in a while were becoming astonishingly more regular, like systemic lupus, fibromyalgia, and Chronic Fatigue Syndrome. I won't even mention the things that won't necessarily kill you, but will certainly alter your quality of life, like fibroid tumors, menopause or the all-too-often under-diagnosed clinical depression.

Even with the dozens of drugs in my PDR (Physicians Desk Reference) and fancy tests to order, I was not even scratching the surface on the preventative end. I was well-trained to fix a problem, but I was not so successful at preventing it from happening …this in the face of patients who were getting increasingly dissatisfied with the health care system and unhappy with the amount of medicine being given to them. (Yet, these patients were unwilling to get to the gym or put down the Newports, fried chicken and Heineken. They had the ability to "Google" anything medical and call it "research" and at the same time looked to me as their physician to "make it better".) I began to think about the correlation between what we eat and how we feel, what we eat and how we

(UNIFICATION)

help (or hinder) the body's God-given ability to heal itself. For quite some time I thought about how good it would be to be able to incorporate sound principles of wellness – as opposed to merely treating illness – into my practice.

Folks, if you remember nothing else I tell you today, remember the power of your thoughts. Guard them carefully and be careful what you wish for. In my case, somewhere in the Universe, someone was listening, and I think because the motive was not selfish, and was for a greater good, I did not have to leave (Grace Family Medical in Brooklyn, NY) for the answer. At the right time and in the right way, two like minds came together with a common goal... to change these dreadful statistics and to snatch back wellness one-person–at-a-time, if necessary. Our project, simply stated, was to gather a group of individuals, partner with them in a wellness program based on holistic strategies....and track their progress over a 12 week period. As a medical person, I would measure simple parameters, such as weight, BMI, blood pressure, lipid levels and diabetic parameters. At the end of the 12 weeks, we would measure and report significant change.

This program has yielded magnificent results, many measurable, and some intangible. Several of the diabetics have seen improvement in their numbers: Two individuals have decreased their medication – one has come off completely. Many of the "hypertensives" have improved; Lipid levels have lowered between 20 and 50 points – this is significant by any scientific parameter. What is even more significant is that whatever it is they did was done without DRUGS, surgery or anything that cannot be duplicated. And that is where the true blessings of this program lie. This has to be reproducible and sustainable. Going forward ...I hope that this transformation continues and that your example will transform others. Statistics are only significant if they stand the test of time. You, *Magnificent Ones* have a made a lifestyle shift. My wish for you is that you defy the odds, shame the numbers. Create those Circles of Wellness and be forever survivors and never statistics.

I have to express my deep personal thanks and affection to my partner in Wellness, Queen Afua. What an honor to be able to call you a Friend as well as a colleague. To Dr. Rita Strickland and her team, my deep gratitude and appreciation. Collecting any amount of medical data is a daunting undertaking, and I could not have done it without you. To Queen Afua's dedicated support staff, it has been a pleasure working with you and learning from you and with you. Life is never the same after your first holistic wellness sweat session or glass of green juice.

It is my wish and desire that all of us go forth and in our own ways do a little something every day to promote wellness, which is more than the mere opposite of illness, first within ourselves, and then with those to whom we come in contact. That in my opinion is the best way to reverse statistics in our lifetime.

Thank you very much.
Dr. Bernadette Sheridan

(UNIFICATION)

It's Time For Change

With hospitals closing…
It's time for change

With health insurance rising…
It's time for change

With toxic, violent, stressed-out families and communities…
It's time for change

With the global health of people of color spiraling down …
It's time for change

With the prison system, mental ward, operating rooms over saturated.
It's time for change

With the rise of sex trafficking and unnecessary hysterectomy.
It's time for change

It's time for We, The People to make the shift; to make the exodus to wellness; the power to heal is within us
How do we make the change? What is the solution?

We must …
Form holistic communities through Circles of Wellness.

We must …
Set our goals and our lifestyles to build Global Circles of Wellness

When do we start?
Activate your Circle now.

Circle will have an impact on the restoration of the wellness of our community!

Break your patterns of distraction.

Use everything you have everything you know to Heal Thyself.
The Time is Now.
"All Power To The People"

(PARADIGM SHIFT 3)

RESTORATION

Cultivating an Emerald Green Lifestyle

"Golden Are My Limbs, Blue My Crown,
Emerald My Body."

from Papyrus of Ani

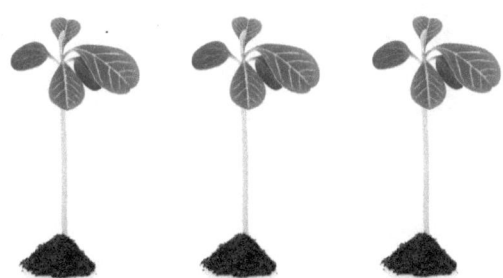

(RESTORATION)

SHIFT TO GREEN

"I am the pure one coming from the green fields."
PAPYRUS OF ANI

Deciding to make the paradigm shift to live an Emerald Green Lifestyle is deciding to embrace optimal and radiant physical, mental, spiritual, relationship and economic well being. Living an Emerald Green Lifestyle is the key to

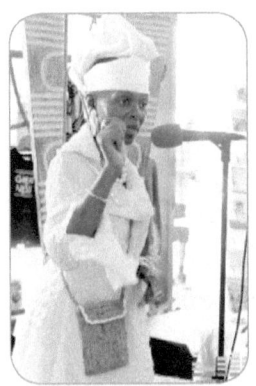

the regeneration of the entire anatomy. Through photosynthesis, sunlight radiates into plants, giving off the green pigmentation called **chlorophyll**, a power substance contained in plant life that restores, repairs, rebuilds, and rejuvenates. To consume of Green Life Formula I is to consume liquid sunlight. Drinking and eating green life that comes from plants restores the brain cells that prevent brain tumors, Alzheimer's and poor memory. Drinking and eating green life that comes from living green plants restores the blood and prevents high and low blood pressure.

Green Life balances the nervous system by preventing stress and memory loss. Green Life repairs skin and soothes suffering eczema, boils and pimples. Green Life restores bones that are arthritic.

By living an Emerald Green Lifestyle you can balance, repair and rejuvenate your relationships. Eating fresh, organic, green – rich leafy salads increases one's communication and listening skills. Drinking and eating green-rich foods has an impact on one's forgiveness capacity and ability to release the past and learn from the experiences for change and transformation. Additionally, the more you saturate the blood tissue cells, the brain and the nervous system with organic green juice and herbs specific to repairing such as Alfalfa, Dandelion and Fennel,

(Crocheted "Green & White Plarn Purse" handmade by GrandMary – 2014)

the closer you get to healing thyself. Continue to say to yourself: "When I choose Emerald Green Live Foods I will improve the qualities that are my tools for harmony in my life and with all my relations."

When my children were young and had to go into the world be in school, on the block, in the community with family, or around strangers, I would saturate their bodies with green juice, green supplements and green foods to protect them from harm. I did this to raise their vibration so high above the norm that they would be out of harm's way. Back then no one believed me, but I was clear we are what we eat and what we attract. Low frequency living keeps children, teenagers, young adults and the elderly in a constant state of harm, violence and disease. We are preyed on by human vultures; we experience dis-ease according to low levels of frequency; our vibration.

Fast Food Generation, BEWARE of flesh food, junk food, sugary substances and food micro-waved into a living hell. Consuming dead, genetically modified, lifeless substances lowers our frequency, leaving us more accessible to violence and abuse. What we ingest creates the environment for what and who we attract to our lives. "Detox your body, mind, soul, words, actions, and relationships from dis-eased living; Come into Emerald Green Living, now, and witness a life shift within yourself, your family, and your community."

(RESTORATION)

How Do I Rejuvenate Myself?

Can I get my wellness back?

Get back your lungs naturally from asthma and other respiratory diseases.

Gain control of your pancreas & save your life when you detoxify from diabetes.

Overcome headaches, depression, and mental health challenges.

Put an end to high blood pressure in your family tree.

Make parenting easier with childhood diseases prevention guidance.

Break the cycle of obesity when you gain control of emotional eating whether day to day to during holiday happenings.

Release stress (even under pressure) with nature's helpers.

Boost your immune system which is the natural protection against wellness challenges from the common cold to STDs .

Women: Save your womb with fibroid prevention techniques.

Men: Empower your prostate holistically for potency

You Can Get Your Wellness Back

Where do I start?

Learn from nuts to sprouts, from A to Z how to detox and rejuvenate your mind, body and spirit.

Learn from A to Z, from nuts to sprouts, how to detox and rejuvenate your mind, body and spirit.

Learn to support your wellness with foods, herbs, elements, attitude, mediation, hydrotherapy, juice therapy, energy work, and vitamin supplements.

Use the five elements to reverse the aging process and restore your life.

You Can Get Your Wellness Back

What steps do I take?

Continue to think: Heal Thyself...

Continue to think Circles of Wellness...

Continue to explore this text, your Passport to Healthy Living

(RESTORATION)

THE 4 PS OF OPTIMAL WELLNESS

- **The Purpose**
  - Be on Purpose.
  - Establish your purpose. *Write your Mission Statement*. Set your goals clearly and attract to yourself optimal wellness in body, mind, and spirit.

- **The Preparation**
  - Prepare Yourself.
  - Choose the holistic dietary program you need to establish for your journey on the road to wellness. Consider seeking the assistance of a wellness consultant for additional guidance on your journey to Optimal Wellness.

- **The Process**
  - Enjoy the Process.
  - Choose a wellness consultant to guide you as you begin transformation of your body, mind and spirit. Enjoy your detox and fortifying process of 21 to 84 days (a season) to secure a lifetime of health and longevity.

- **The Prosperity**
  - Attract Prosperity.
  - Manifest the first 3 Ps, in order to gain the fourth "P"– prosperity. Your harvest will be a healthy mind, a healthy body, and a vibrant spirit. Prosperity in these circles will attract a prosperous life.

---

* Write your Mission Statement. Write down your thoughts about the 4Ps in your life. Examine how the 4 Ps are related to each other in your Circle of Self. List goals you wish to achieve. List strategies you will use to achieve those goals. From your lists, create a Mission Statement to remind yourself of your goals and your plans for becoming a balanced, prosperous and complete Circle of Self.

9 Steps To Holistic Living
(How to make a stress-free transition to a toxin-free way of life)

1. **Drink** herbal formulas for 7 to 21 days. The amount of herbs and water will vary for each participant.
2. **Avoid fried foods** which can contribute to heart attacks, high blood pressure and strokes. Instead, eat vegetables steamed 3 to 5 minutes. *(Nearly one in three US adults has high blood pressure. Since there are no symptoms, nearly one-third of those patients have undiagnosed high blood pressure for years. Undiagnosed, and therefore untreated and uncontrolled high blood pressure, can lead to stroke, heart attack, heart failure, and/or kidney failure. www.americanheart.org)*
3. **Replace dairy products** which contribute to respiratory ills (asthma, bronchitis and hay fever). Instead, obtain proteins and calcium from seed or nut milk and green vegetable juices. *(Today, more than 35 million Americans are living with diseases such as asthma, emphysema and bronchitis. www.lungusa.org)*
4. **Avoid Sugar** (brown or white) which contributes to arthritis, tooth decay, stress, depression, mood swings and acne. Enjoy, instead **soaked** dried fruits (currants, raisins, dates, apricots.) *(Processed sugar is deadly. It suppresses the immune system's ability to manufacture antibodies. Sugar depletes the B vitamins needed to detoxify the liver, the most important organ in the body-healing process. www.stopcancer.com)*
5. **Drink 8 glasses of water daily** to prevent dehydration, premature aging and constipation. *(Dehydration is loss of water and the blood salts (potassium and sodium). Extreme dehydration damages the kidneys, brain and heart.)*
6. **Drink Green.** A pint of green juice daily helps prevent sluggishness, poor circulation, obesity, cellulite and brittle bones. *(According to the 1999-2000 National Health & Nutrition Examination Survey (NHANES), more than 64% of US adults are either overweight or obese.)*

(RESTORATION)

7. **Reduce weekly animal flesh** consumption to half of your present intake. Replace extremely difficult-to-digest animal flesh proteins (pork, beef, lamb, etc.) with skinless organic chicken and fish (with scales; no shellfish). Better still; eat vegetable proteins (beans, peas, lentils, sprouts). For optimal digestion eat proteins only at mid-day. Make changes to help minimize and/or prevent cancer, hypertension, constipation and poor circulation. *(Digesting meat depletes enzymes that are critical to the immune system for fighting cancer cells. Vegetable proteins don't use up those enzymes.)*

8. **Eat salad.** Two servings daily of vegetables, steamed, in salad, soup or broth supports colon wellness and rejuvenation. Enjoy 1 to 2 servings of fresh fruit for internal body purity and to prevent sinus congestion, hay fever, colds.

9. **Listen** to the Empowerment CDs or read the techniques to begin aligning your inner body to wellness.*

---

* Empowerment CDs to assist you in you in your journey to wellness are available at Queen Afua Wellness Store.
Please visit www.queenafua.com.

84 Day Whole Living Program

The goal of the Circle of Wellness program is to bring family and friends with you as you journey within the FOUR levels of detoxification. The mission to purify, detoxify and unify will strengthen you and all of your relationships. Your Circles of Wellness can be a catalyst which aids the recovery of self, the people and the planet. We can move from being disease-infested to being a holistic, purified people living in harmony with natureand with one another. As we honor and respect ourselves, we will honor and respect nature. We will be protecting our inner and outer environments. Let us create a vibrant humanity as we create pure water, pure air and rejuvenated soil for a healthy Earth. In this way, the Circles of Wellness and The City of Wellness will converge at the universal levels of High Living.

Usually, all four levels of wellness will coexist within a collective Circle of Wellness. Each one in the circle seeking a holistic lifestyle will study by reading **Heal Thyself for Health & Longevity** and **The City of Wellness: Restoring Your Health Through the 7 Kitchens of Consciousness.** The tools for wellness and therapeutic applications listed below are used during all four levels of detoxification.

Tools for wellness:
- Green Life Formula I (aids the immune system) - added to juices – taken 3x, daily
- Master Herbal Formula II* (aids prevention of cysts & tumors in the body) – taken weekly
- Woman's Life Formula VII * (aids strengthening female reproductive organs) – taken weekly
- Manpower Formula VIII* (aids strengthening male reproductive organs) – taken weekly
- Colon Ease Formula III (for flushing the kidneys and the liver) –taken weekly

- Herbal Laxatives Formula IV (aids waste elimination) – taken in the evenings, weekly
- Breath of Life Formula VI (aids mucus elimination) –3 drops taken 1–2x, daily

Therapeutic applications:
- Enemas (remove toxins from colon) – done personally, 2 - 3x weekly
- Colonics (more thorough removal of wastes from colon) – done by health practitioner, 2 - 8x per season based on individual wellness level
- Salt or herbal baths (for relaxing and relieving stress) taken 3 - 4x weekly
- Exercise (full body benefits) stretch, walk, do yoga, etc. at least 30 minutes, daily
- Warm water (to flush impurities) – eight glasses, daily
- Rejuvenation Clay Formula V (aids swollen/painful areas of the body) – applications as needed.

---

* During the second 21 Day cycle, the Master Herbal Formula tonics will be replaced by the Woman's Life Herbal Formula or Man's Life Herbal Formula, according to gender and taken as needed. For cycles 3 and 4, the Master Herbal Formula will be alternated with Woman's Life Formula or Man's Life Formula, accordingly.

LET'S DO THE MATH
Self Diagnosis through Foods

Toxic Foods	Daily: # of servings	Weekly: # of Daily x 7 =	Monthly: # of Weekly x 4 =	Yearly: # of Monthly x12 =	Lifetime: # of Yearly x Age =
Meat Intake Pork, beef, lamb, chicken, goat, fish, etc.					
Dairy Intake Milk, cheese, ice-cream, eggs, butter, yogurt, etc.					
Starch Intake White rice, white bread, white potatoes					
Sugar Intake Corn syrup, fructose, brown & white sugar					

The 1st Step to Making a Dietary Paradigm Shift

Use the chart above to calculate the number of times you have consumed various toxic foods. Total your *daily, weekly, monthly* and *annual* toxic intake. Based on the chart you can do the calculations to determine what has caused your current wellness challenges. You can begin to answer the question: *Why do I suffer from dis-eases?* As you begin to change your Dietary Lifestyle, ultimately you will change your conditions of did-ease to states of wellness for your body, mind and spirit.

Self Diagnosis through Foods (cont)

Related Disease	Related Emotions	Related Needs	Wellness Alternative
Numbing sensation in extremities; hypertension; cancer in: reproductive organs (male and female), colon, throat, etc.; kidney failure, toxic sperm (men), toxic womb (women)	Anger, Rage, Aggression	Seeking contentment and inner peace	TVP beans, lentils, sprouts, raw nuts and seeds, Green Life Formula I
Fibroids, constipation, clogged arteries, respiratory issues, asthma, shortness of breath, colds, hay fever, allergies, toxic/acidic sperm,	Disappointment, hurt	Seeking Mother love and Father love; being nursed, supported	Almond milk, sesame milk, green vegetable juice
Constipation, abdominal bloating, gas, shortness of breath, distended colon	Stagnation, emptiness, entrapment	Seeking fulfillment to move forward	Sprouted bread, brown rice, couscous, bulgur wheat, tabouli, buckwheat pancakes
Stress, diabetes, headaches, arthritis, hip replacement, depression, mood swings, devitalized & weak sperm	Depression, temper, mood swings	Seeking love, satisfaction, contentment, human kindness	Licorice root, raw honey, dates, raisins, currants, agave, Stevia

Transformation for Wellness
You have created dis-ease by 20, 30, 80 years of toxic eating.
Now, you can create wellness by living an Emerald Green lifestyle

Dietary Lifestyles And Nutrition Kitchen Meal Plans

Level 1 – Beginner – Energized Flexitarian

Shift to Energized Flexitarian: Right now you eat meats, cooked foods and other foods that do not entirely support your wellness. Your transition from these choices can lead to an increased level of wellness. Begin by eating easier to digest organic chicken and fish (with scales; no shellfish). Eventually omit flesh foods (beef, pork, lamb, goat, turkey, chicken, and fish). Incorporate into your diet: whole grains, sprouts, beans, peas, and lentils (soaked in water overnight). Consume vegetable protein. Eat greater amounts of fresh fruits and vegetables. Use Natural and Whole Foods to prepare favorite family recipes.

Notes:
1. Maintain a 30 minute break between eating and drinking for optimal digestion of meal
2. Take 1-2 oz. of Wheatgrass 3-7 times a week with 12-16 oz. of water.
3. Eat animal protein midday between 12-4PM only. (Animal protein: steamed fish (no shellfish) or 1 piece baked organic chicken with skin removed).
4. When the sun goes down, do not eat proteins or starches. Eat only fruits & salads.

	Energized Flexitarian
Upon Rising: Pre-Breakfast	Kidney Liver Flush: Juice of 1 lemon, (not if you have HBP) 1 pinch of cayenne pepper, 1-2 Tbs. Inner-Colon Ease, 1-2 garlic cloves or 12 drops of Kyolic in 8 oz. of warm H2O. Blend, shake or stir.
BF: (Before liquid breakfast)	Master Herbal Tea or Woman's Life Tea or Man's Life Tea 8-12 oz. (previously steeped overnight)
Liquid Breakfast 7:00	1-2 Tbs. Green Life added to 12-16 oz. of H2O OR 12-16 oz. fresh squeezed juice mixed with H2O
Solid Breakfast 7:30	Citrus Fruit Platter: oranges, grapefruits, pineapples & lemons; OR Sub acid Fruit Platter: apples, pears, plums, peaches, cherries & berries ; OR Melon Platter: honeydew & cantaloupe; OR , watermelon (best If eaten alone); OR Tropical Fruit Platter: mangos & papayas ; OR Optional: whole grain cereal with almond or sesame milk; OR spelt or whole grain pancakes or waffles
Liquid Lunch 12:00	Juice ½ Cup each: Kale, String Beans, Cabbage added to 1-2 T Green Life in 12-16 oz. of water Add 1-2 Tbs. Green Life Formula Wheatgrass 1-2 oz. 3-7 x a week with 12-16 oz. of H2O

Energized Flexitarian (cont.)	
Solid Lunch **12:30**	50% Salad Live Greens : asparagus w/ dandelion greens 30% Steamed Veggies: mustard greens w/pearl onions OR vegetable broth or soup. 10%-20% Starch: soaked couscous w/sunflower seeds & spike seasonings 10%-20% Protein: baked organic chicken (skinless) or organic BBQ tofu w/cajun seasonings
Liquid Dinner **6:00**	Repeat lunch vegetable juice, and add 1-2 T Green Life to 12-16 oz. H2O
Solid Dinner **6:30**	50% Live Green Salad: escarole, kale w/red pepper 30% steamed veggies: curry cauliflower 10%-20% Starch: millet, couscous, bulgur wheat, brown or black rice 10%-20% Vegan protein

Level 2 – Intermediate— Super Vegetarian

Shift to Super Vegetarian: Consume only vegetarian foods. Omit all flesh foods (seafood, beef, pork, lamb, turkey, goat, etc.). Fresh vegetable intake should include 50% –75% live food and 50% –25% vegetables. Steam vegetables lightly to retain maximum live enzymes and oxygen.

Super Vegetarian	
Upon Rising: Pre-Breakfast	Kidney Liver Flush: Juice of 1 lemon, (not if you have HBP) 1 pinch of cayenne pepper, 1-2Tbs. Inner-Colon Ease, 1-2 garlic cloves or 12 drops of Kyolic in 8 oz. of warm H2O. Blend, shake or stir.
BF: (Before liquid breakfast)	Master Herbal Tea or Woman's Life Tea or Man's Life Tea 8-12 oz. (previously steeped overnight)
Liquid Breakfast 7:00	Blueberry & Blackberry Juice w/ 1-2Tbs. Green Life Formula
Solid Breakfast 7:30	Blueberries w/blended pears sprinkled w/shredded coconut. OR Blueberries w/blue corn cereal & almond milk
Liquid Lunch 12:00	Juice of celery 2 stalks, ½ cup each of broccoli and chard ½ cup. Add 1-2 Tbs. Green Life Wheatgrass 1-2 oz. 3-7 x a week with 12-16 oz. of H2O
Solid Lunch 12:30	50% –75% Salad Live Greens: Romaine lettuce w/shredded broccoli; steamed zucchini Protein Sources: Choose from T.V.P. Soya Curry Chicken or Beans, Peas, Lentils, Raw Sprouted Nuts (soaked overnight)
Liquid Dinner 6:00	Wheatgrass 2-4 oz. OR 1-2 Tbs. Green Life in 12-16 oz. of water
Solid Dinner 6:30	Salad Steamed veggies, whole grain brown rice; Veggie Protein: Black bean soup

REMINDERS:

Vegetarian Protein Choices:

Beans, Peas, Lentils, Raw Soaked Nuts, Raw Soaked Seeds, Sprouts, Spirulina

Sweeteners:

Use Soaked Dates, Raisins or Currents.

Level 3 – Advanced Radiant Raw Vegan

Shift to Advanced Radiant Raw Vegan: Consume 100% live, uncooked food. Live foods include organic live proteins (sprouted beans, raw soaked nuts and seeds, avocadoes), salads, live soups, uncooked grains such as couscous, tabouli, bulgur wheat. Consume whole or juiced fresh fruits and vegetables. Start your day with 8 oz. of Kidney-Liver Flush. Throughout the morning, before noon complete 5 cups of Master Herbal or Woman's Life Herbal (women) or Man's Life Herbal (men). Throughout the day drink a ½ gallon of warm water (8 oz. glasses).

Advanced Radiant Raw Vegan	
Upon Rising: Pre-Breakfast	Kidney Liver Flush: Juice of 1 lemon, (not if you have HBP) 1 pinch of cayenne pepper, 1-2 Tbs. Inner-Colon Ease, 1-2 garlic cloves or 12 drops of Kyolic in 8 oz. of warm H2O. Blend, shake or stir.
BF: (Before liquid breakfast)	Master Herbal Tea or Woman's Life Tea or Man's Life Tea 8-12 oz. (previously steeped overnight)
Liquid Breakfast 7:00	8 oz. Unsweetened Cranberry Juice w/1-2 Tbs. Green Life
Solid Breakfast 7:30	Diced pears w/blueberries strawberries OR raspberries. Slice fruit and blend to a sauce. Pumpkin seed: Soak ½ cup of soaked pumpkin seeds (Recommended for the prostate.)
Liquid Lunch 12:00	For Blood Restoration: ½ cup kale, ½ cup chard, 1-2 red radishes, ¼ cup ginger root, ½ beet and 2 Tbs. Green Life. Wheatgrass 1-2 oz. 3-7 x a week with 12-16 oz. of H2O
Solid Lunch 12:30	Green Salad: Grated beets & red peppers Veggies: 1 cup raw okra with olive oil, sprinkled with Spike seasoning; Mock tuna wrapped in lettuce leaves OR seaweed wrapped in lettuce leaves or additional seaweed Protein: Add mung bean, radish, or ½ cup broccoli sprouts over mock tuna or salad
Liquid Dinner 6:00	2 – 4 oz. Wheatgrass OR 1-2 Tbs. Green Life in 12-16 oz. of water

Advanced Radiant Raw Vegan (cont.)	
Solid Dinner **6:30**	Live Green Salad: spinach, mung beans and raw soaked nuts or seeds
	Steamed Veggies: Live okra or broccoli dish
	Live Starch: Soaked couscous, bulgur etc.
	Protein: ½ avocado or ½ cup almonds, filberts

REMINDERS:

(Also see Food As Medicine in this chapter)

Vegetarian Protein Choices:

Beans, Peas, Lentils, Raw Soaked Nuts, Raw Soaked Seeds, Sprouts, Spirulina

Sweeteners:

Use Soaked Dates, Raisins or Currents.

Level 4 – Purified Juiceatarian (Advanced Therapeutic Juice Fast)

Shift to Purified Juiceatarian: Consume 100% organic liquid meals only. This is usually only done for specific periods of time as a cleansing regime. An advanced cleaning regime consists of two vegetable juice meals for rejuvenation and one fruit juice meal for detoxification, daily. Additionally, there should be a daily intake of a ½ gallon of warm water (8 oz. glasses), 5 cups Master Herbal tea and 8 oz. of Kidney-Liver flush.

LEVEL 4 is a therapeutic juice fast that should be followed for (7) seven days each season (84 days) Elements of the juice fast are part of all four steps.

Purified Juiceatarian	
Upon Rising: Pre-Breakfast	Kidney Liver Flush: Juice of 1 lemon, (not if you have HBP) 1 pinch of cayenne pepper, 1-2 Tbs. Inner-Colon Ease, 1-2 garlic cloves or 12 drops of Kyolic in 8 oz. of warm H2O. Blend, shake or stir.
BF: (Before liquid breakfast)	Master Herbal Tea or Woman's Life Tea or Man's Life Tea 8-12. The night before boil 3-4 cups of water. Turn off flame and add 3-4 Tbs. of Herbal Formula to hot water. Let steep overnight, then strain in the morning. Drink from sunrise; finish before midday.
Liquid Breakfast 7:00	Fresh Organic Fruit Juice choices: Acidic fruits: orange, grapefruit, tangerine, pineapples; OR Melons: watermelon, cantaloupe, honeydew melon; OR Sub Acidic: apples, pears, plums, peaches, berries; OR Tropical: papaya & mangos; OR Combine 8 oz. of fresh-pressed juice with 12-16 oz. of water & 1 Tbs. Green Life. Drink once a day
Before Liquid Lunch 12:00	Wheatgrass 2-4 oz. OR 1-2 Tbs. Green Life in 12-16 oz. of water
Liquid Lunch 12:30	Green Juice choices: 12-16 oz. juice with 16 oz. of water. cucumber, watercress, & parsley; OR turnip, broccoli & kale; OR celery, chard & string beans Combine 12-16 oz. juice with 16 oz. of water. Drink twice a day.

Purified Juiceatarian (cont.)	
Liquid Dinner **6:00**	Repeat Liquid Lunch: Green Juice choices: 12-16 oz. juice with 16 oz. of water. cucumber, watercress, & parsley; OR turnip, broccoli & kale ; OR celery, chard & string beans Combine 12-16 oz. juice with 16 oz. of water. Drink twice a day.

Brain Food

One more thing about food is the importance of feeding the brain. Even before conception, both potential parents who are considering having children should give yourselves 1- 4 seasons (12 weeks) of detox from toxic substances to prevent passing toxicity through the blood and DNA down to your potential fetus. In addition to eliminating the use of drugs, alcohol and cigarettes, detox from flesh food which contributes to cancerous cell growth, dairy which contributes to respiratory blockage i.e. asthma and allergies. Refrain from consuming white flour products which lead to constipation. Refrain from sugar which contributes to depression and potential suicidal thoughts, as well as brain deformities that can lead to Autism in babies and Alzheimer's symptoms in the elderly. Consuming sugar is as dangerous as taking crack; crack is a derivative of cocaine. Sugar is only a few molecules away from cocaine. The complex challenge with sugar is that it is a legal "drug" and that most prepackaged foods are saturated with sugar. "Consumer Beware."

Parents, you can detox your blood from sugar craving with the bitter herbs available in Master Herbal Formula II for at least 21 days. (Add 4 tsp. of Formula II to 4 C of water, steep overnight, strain and drink in the morning.) Replace sugar with a family fruit bowl. Help your children replace processed sweets, candy and junk foods with whole foods such as apples, pears, plums, oranges, berries and grapes. Stop feeding fast food to your children. Fast food clogs, blocks, poisons, and decays our children's brains and bodies. Set up your Nutrition Kitchen Pharmacy. Encourage family participation as you create and prepare meals in your Nutrition Kitchen with your children. Easily prepared dinner meals include salads and salad dressings, steamed veggies, veggie soups, whole grains and vegetable protein dishes. For breakfast the family can prepare fruit, cereal or porridge blended with apples, pears or papaya and topped with berries. To maximize brain power prepare fruit smoothies and add 1 Tbs. of Green Life Formula I to smoothies or to fresh pressed fruit juice.

"Supa Brain" Reminders

Parents it is never too late. Start creating a "Supa Brain" with your child in order to rejuvenate and protect your youth.

Step 1
Prevent eating sugar. It is s a drug that destroys the brain cells and as a result contributes to ADD, depression, violence, hyperactivity and mood swings in children and teens.

Step 2
Encourage your child (and your family) to eat live 1-2 x a day. Instead of junk food and fast food, eat vegetables and salads.

Step 3
Give your child 4-8 oz. of vegetable juice, daily.

Step 4
Add (1 – 2 Tbs.) Green Life Formula I to fresh breakfast juice of fresh grapefruit or orange or apple or pear juice. Follow juice with 8-16 oz. of H2O.

Step 5
Invert for the brain. Have your child invert daily. Before getting out of bed in the morning or going to sleep in the evening have your child lie down flat in the bed. Place 3 pillows, one on top of the next. Then have your child place their legs over the pillows and rest in that position for 10 minutes. This will promote greater oxygen flow and blood circulation to the brain and nervous system.

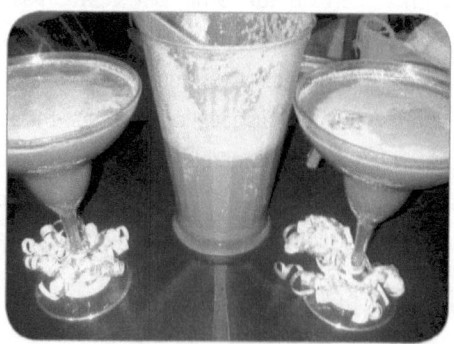

(RESTORATION)

PREPARE FOR YOUR JOURNEY

Before you begin detoxification and purification...
If you are presently consulting a physician for existing health challenges, CONTINUE to follow the advice of your physician. The information provided herein is designed is to be inspirational and help you make informed decisions about your health. Neither this material nor the program is intended to be a substitute for medical advice and treatment that has been prescribed by your doctor.

Officially begin your 7-Day, 21 Day or 12-Week Wellness Program on a **Monday.** Use the days before you begin to prepare your body, mind, spirit, and environment for your exciting journey to wellness.

Some things to do:
- **Purchase the holistic foods and herbs you will need.**
- **Prepare your Nutrition Kitchen Pharmacy.**

    You will need:
    - A juicer to juice live fruits and vegetables
    - A blender to blend juices and nutrients
    - A stainless steel pot for preparing herbal teas

- **Prepare your Hydrotherapy Room (bathroom).**

    You will need:
    - A footstool - raises feet and knees to facilitate elimination
    - An enema bag to assist colon cleansing while detoxing

- **Prepare for your physical fitness.**

    You will need:
    - Sneakers and loose fitting clothing
    - Yoga mat

- **Prepare your mind.**

    Read material on wellness such as, *Heal Thyself for Health & Longevity and The*

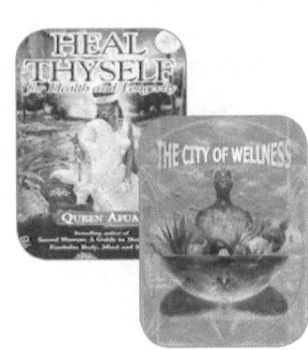

City of Wellness: Restoring Your Health Through the 7 Kitchens of Consciousness. This is also a good time to meditate and think about goals you would like to accomplish while you are on your journey to wellness.

- **Prepare your spirit.**

    Consider the mantra and affirmation below. Look for others that are appropriate for you and your goals.

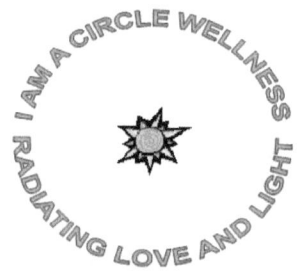

AFFIRMATION

I am on my pathway to wellness.
I am on my pathway to self love and healing.
I am on my pathway to transformation.
I am on my pathway to
CIRCLES OF WELLNESS.
Through Circles of Wellness
I am restoring WHOLENESS.

- **Prepare to record your journey to wellness.**

    Purchase or prepare a notebook to record your transformation experiences of body, mind and spirit. Use the charts as guides for preparing your Wellness Journal.

Say It Is So
(Affirmations)

Write down these affirmations. Choose and recite the affirmation(s) appropriate to your purpose, especially during days of detox and purification.

1. **I have entered** a Circle of Wellness, doorway to The City of Wellness.
2. **I commit to living** a holistic, rejuvenated life that will empower me.
3. **I am overcoming** toxic attitudes of my past, with a patient calm spirit and an open heart.
4. **I am going forward** towards wellness. I will not be turned back to toxicity.
5. **I am lovingly consuming** whole foods from nature's pharmacy in order to transform my body into a living temple of wellness.
6. **I am relentlessly rejuvenating** my body, mind and spirit in order to raise my wellness frequency.
7. **I am filled with gratitude** for the healing that is being manifested in my Circle of Wellness.
8. **I am nurturing** my new-found relationship with myself.
9. **I am nurturing** a newfound relationship with nature.
10. **I am embracing** healthy relationships; together we will build Circles of Wellness.
11. **I am claiming** my right to live a peace-filled life within a Circle of Wellness.
12. **I celebrate** my entry into a Circle of Wellness.
13. **I am releasing away** past pain and resentment.
14. **I accept** peace, power, wellness and joy into my life.
15. **I am detoxing** my life of hurt, fear, and resentment.
16. **I am embracing** my wellness to reconnect to my natural beauty.

17. **I release** anger and all symptoms of dis-ease; I embrace wellness for my body, mind, and spirit.
18. **I am learning** to nurture my self-tranquility for my wellness.
19. **I am soothing** my spirit by removing hurt, fear, and resentment, and di s-ease from my life.
20. **I embrace** my wellness. My destiny is liberation! I am free!
21. **I am rejuvenating** my body, mind and spirit into wholeness, health, and happiness

(RESTORATION)

WRITE ON
(DAILY JOURNAL)

Week beginning _____

Affirmation of the week: _____

Goal for the week: _____

_____

Rejuvenation Monday _____

_____

_____

_____

_____

_____

Vibrant Tuesday _____

_____

_____

_____

_____

_____

(CIRCLES OF WELLNESS)

Power Wednesday

Radiant Thursday

Detox Friday

(Restoration)

Fortification Saturday _____

_____

_____

_____

_____

_____

Wellness Sunday _____

_____

_____

_____

_____

_____

Reflections on goal of the week _____

_____

_____

_____

_____

_____

(CIRCLES OF WELLNESS)

CHECK UP
(DAILY CHECKLIST)

Week beginning _____

	Date	Date	Date	Date	Date	Date	Date
SUNRISE							
1. Circle of Wellness meditation between the hours of 4 AM—6 AM							
2. Pre-Breakfast: Kidney-Liver Flush/ Colon Ease Formula. Drink 3 glasses warm H2O w/ juice of 1 lemon or lime							
3. Daily Exercise: Power walk							
4a. Liquid Breafast: Fruit Juice w/2 Tbs. GL							
4b. Solid Breakfast: Fruit platter							
5. Herbal Formula 3t to 3 cups. Drink daily before 1PM							
MIDDAY							
6a. Liquid Lunch: 16 oz. Green Juice w/2 Tbs. Green Life							

6b. Solid Lunch: steamed vegetables, green salad w/vegetable protein								
7. Write in Circle of Wellness Journal								
8. Share wellness with someone else								
SUNSET								
9a. Liquid Dinner: 16 oz. Green Juice 2 Tbs. Green Life								
9b. Solid Dinner: steamed vegetables, green salad w/vegetable protein								
10. Listen daily to Empowerment CD (one for each day of the week)								
11. Colon wellness: Take herbal laxatives 3 x, weekly and enemas 3x weekly								
12. Full Body Bath: 2 - 4 lbs Epsom Salt or 1-2 lbs Dead Sea Salt, morning or night. NO SALTS if you have high blood pressure. Use apple cider vinegar (2 Tbs. -1 cup) instead of salt.								

(PARADIGM SHIFT 4)

EMPOWERMENT

Using Wellness Tools

"All Power to the People"

Unity chant from The 1960s Civil Rights Movement

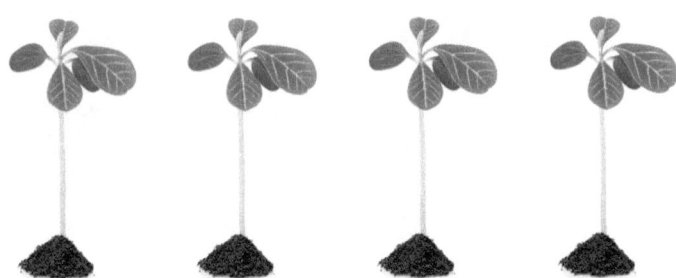

(EMPOWERMENT)

ELEMENTS AND WHEELS AND FORMULAS

Empowerment Tools for Wellness

Air, Fire, Water, and Earth are the elements that make up our bodies and make up Nature and are a part of the Universe. We are one from the microcosmic to the macrocosmic. We are on one planet feeding and warming ourselves from the same sun (fire); inhaling vitality from the same atmosphere (air). We drink and bathe from the same waters (ocean, lakes, falls, and rivers) and obtain our nourishment from the same Earth (trees, plants, flowers and clay). Everything we need to Heal Thyself is within the elements. When we are aligned with the elements, we are aligned with health and vitality in body, mind and spirit. In Radionic holistic energy readings, a tool called the pendulum is used to pick up ("read") our energy field. A seasoned pendulum energy reader is trained to interpret the direction in which the pendulum swings and determine one's vibrational frequency, which indicates one's states of disease or well being. When we are toxic and out of alignment our energy vibration will cause the pendulum to rotate in a counter-clockwise direction If we are living in alignment with Nature our energy vibration will cause the pendulum to rotate in a clockwise direction which indicates that we are in a state of wellness, harmony and unity with ourselves and all our relations.

Within the Paradigm Shift Chapter are tools you can use for yourself and your family. You can begin by using the wellness Intake Chart to help you to identify the problems and challenges to your wellness of body, mind and spirit. Once you have identified the challenges you are better empowered to take the steps to realign yourself with the flow of yourself and the flow of Nature and the Universe. The second worksheet is a list of suggestions for using the Queen Afua Wellness Formulas and Products to address over one hundred wellness challenges.

Finally, there are the 12 Wellness Empowerment Circles (formerly called Wellness Empowerment Wheels) that have been in Queen Afua's Heal Thyself 'tool-kit' and available to her clients for at least two decades. (See following Assessment and Product Usage Charts.)

Study, reflect and apply the recommendations, guides and charts in this chapter to harmonize yourself to wholeness. Maintain the holistic lifestyle presented for a minimum of 21 days. If you continue for a maximum of 12 weeks you can reach optimal wellness. The following strategies and recommendations are hands on guides to using the elements for wellness restoration.

On each Wellness Empowerment Circle Wheel are suggestions for drinking Herbal Tonics.

- The recipe for preparing an herbal tonic is: Steep 1 tsp. of each suggested herb in 1 C. of H20 to each tsp. of herb used.
- Instead, one can drink Master Herbal Formula II, unless otherwise advised. (Check with Queen Afua or a Wellness Practitioner if MH2 is appropriate for usage with your wellness challenge).
- Also available are prepared Circle Wellness Tonics at the Queen Afua Wellness Center.
- Finally, always recommended is consultation with Queen Afua or a Wellness Practitioner at the Queen Afua Wellness Center.

Throughout your healing journey record in your journal your challenges, lessons and progress in your quest for Optimal Wellness. Then write in your journal and process on your journey to 360°, complete Circle of Self Wellness.

(EMPOWERMENT)

WELLNESS CHALLENGES CHECKLIST

Please check the following issues as related to your wellness. Some conditions overlap and may be repeated in multiple categories:

General:
- ❑ Blood Pressure-High
- ❑ Blood Pressure-Low
- ❑ Cancer
- ❑ Chronic Pain
- ❑ Diabetes
- ❑ Dizziness
- ❑ Enlarged Thyroid
- ❑ Fainting
- ❑ Fatigue
- ❑ Headaches
- ❑ Hernia
- ❑ Loss of Sleep
- ❑ Pain Over Heart
- ❑ Spitting up Blood
- ❑ Varicose Veins
- ❑ Vomiting
- ❑ Weight Gain
- ❑ Weight Loss

Circulatory:
- ❑ Hardening of Arteries
- ❑ Numbness

Colon/Digestive:
- ❑ Colitis
- ❑ Colon Trouble
- ❑ Constipation
- ❑ Diarrhea
- ❑ Difficult Digestion
- ❑ Distended Abdomen
- ❑ Gas
- ❑ Hemorrhoids

Eyes, Ears, Nose & Throat:
- ❑ Allergies
- ❑ Asthma
- ❑ Colds
- ❑ Earache
- ❑ Eye Pain
- ❑ Gum Trouble
- ❑ Hay Fever
- ❑ Hoarseness
- ❑ Nasal Obstruction
- ❑ Nose Bleeds
- ❑ Sinus Infection
- ❑ Sore Throat
- ❑ Tonsillitis

Heart/Cardio:
- ❑ Heart Attack
- ❑ Heart Disease
- ❑ Rapid Heart Beat
- ❑ Pain Over Heart

Kidney/ Urinary & Genitals:
- ❑ Bedwetting
- ❑ Frequent Urination
- ❑ Genital Dryness
- ❑ Kidney Infection or Stones
- ❑ Painful Urination
- ❑ Swelling Of Ankles
- ❑ Tumors

Emotional/Mental:
- ❑ Alcoholism
- ❑ Depression
- ❑ Nervousness
- ❑ Drug Addiction
- ❑ Eating Disorder
- ❑ Excessive Hunger
- ❑ Emotional Eating

Muscle & Joint:
- ❑ Arthritis
- ❑ Bursitis
- ❑ Foot Trouble
- ❑ Hardening of Arteries
- ❑ Low Back Pain
- ❑ Neck Pain & Stiffness

(CIRCLES OF WELLNESS)

❏ Poor Posture
❏ Spinal Curvature

Nerves:
❏ Epilepsy
❏ Stroke

Respiratory:
❏ Chest Pain
❏ Difficulty Breathing
❏ Emphysema
❏ Spitting up Phlegm
❏ Wheezing
❏ Emphysema

Skin:
❏ Allergies
❏ Boils
❏ Bruises
❏ Cold Sores

❏ Dryness
❏ Eczema
❏ Itching
❏ Measles

Apply to Women:
❏ Cysts
❏ Fibroid Tumors
❏ Incontinence
❏ Vaginal Discharge
❏ Vaginal Itch
❏ Lumps in Breast
❏ # of days of menstrual flow?
_____

❏ Irregular cycle
❏ Cramps
❏ Painful Menstruation
❏ Excessive Menstrual

❏ Bleeding
❏ Infertility
❏ Miscarriage
　❏ Yes ❏ No
If yes, how many?
_____

❏ Hot Flashes
❏ Other Menopausal Symptoms
❏ Hysterectomy

Applied to Men:
❏ Blocked prostate tubes
❏ Burning
❏ Discharge
❏ Incontinence
❏ Infertility
❏ Other Prostate Issues

Indicate any other health concerns or conditions:

_____

_____

_____

_____

_____

(See: *Now That You Know* at the end of the last chapter for the progress percentage monitor list.)

(EMPOWERMENT)

WELLNESS PRODUCT USAGE CHART

Wellness Issue	Product Usage	Wellness Issue	Product Usage	Wellness Issue	Product Usage
Alcoholism	G1, M2	Eczema	G1, M2, C5	Low Blood Pressure	G1, M2
Allergy	G1, M2, B6	Emphysema	G1, M2, L4, B6	Nervousness	G1, M2, B6
Anemia	G1, M2	Epileptic Attack **911**	G1, M2, L4, B6	Numbness	G1, M2, C5, B6
Cancer	G1, M2, L4, C5	Excessive Hunger	G1, L4	Pain Over Heart	G1, M2, L4
Chest Pain	M2, C5	Fainting	G1, M2, B6	Pneumonia	G1, M2, L4, C5
Chronic Pain	M2, C5	Fatigue	G1, M2, B6	Polio	G1, M2, L4, C5
Cold Sores	G1, M2, C5	Gas	G1, L4, CE3	Rapid Heart Beat **911**	G1, M2, L4
Colitis	CE2, L4	Hardening of Arteries	G1, M2	Spitting Up Blood **911**	G1, M2, L4, C5
Colon Trouble	CE3, L4	Headache	G1, M2, L4, B6	Spitting Up Phlegm	B6
Constipation	CE3, L4	Heart Disease	G1, M2, L4, B6	Stroke	G1, M2, L4, C5
Depression	G1, M2, L4	Hemorrhoids	G1, L4	Swelling of Ankles	G1, M2, L4, C5
Diabetes	G1, M2, L4	High Blood Pressure	G1	Ulcers	G1, M2, L4, C5
Diarrhea	CE3, L4	HIV/AIDS	G1, M2, L4, C5 & * (WL7) or (ML8)	STDs / Venereal Disease	G1, M2, L4, C5 & * (WL7) or (ML8)

(147)

(CIRCLES OF WELLNESS)

Wellness Issue	Product Usage	Wellness Issue	Product Usage	Wellness Issue	Product Usage
Difficult Breathing **911**	G1, B6	Infertility	G1, C3, L4, C5 & *(WL7) or (ML8)	Vomiting	G1, L4
Difficult Digestion	CE3, L4	Loss of Sleep	G1, M2	Wheezing	B6
Distention of Abdomen	G1, L4	Loss of Weight	G1, M2		
Bruise Easily	G1, M2, L4, C5	Bursitis	C5	Snore	B6

SKIN	Product Usage	MUSCLE & JOINT	Product Usage	SLEEP & ENERGY LEVELS	Product Usage
Boils	G1, M2, L4, C5	Arthritis	G1, M2, L4, C5	Sleep with mouth open	B6
Bruise Easily	G1, M2, L4, C5	Bursitis	C5	Snore	B6
		Neck Pain & Stiffness	C5	Frequent Urination	ML8, C5
		Spinal Curvature	C5	Impotency	ML8, G1, M2, C5, L4
				Prostate cancer	ML8, G1, M2, C5, L4

(148)

LIFE HEALER – THE POWER TO HEAL IS WITHIN

EYES, EARS, NOSE, THROAT	Product Usage	GENITO/ URINARY	Product Usage	WOMEN ONLY	Women: Alternate M2 to WL7 every 21 days
Asthma	G1, M2, L4, C5, B6	Bedwetting	G1, M2, L4, C5	Cramps	G1, CE3, L4, C5, WL7
Colds	G1, M2, L4, C5, B6	Dryness	CE3	Cysts	G1, CE3, L4, C5, WL7
Ear Ache	G1, M2, L4, C5, B6	Frequent Urination	G1, M2, L4	Hot Flashes	G1, CE3, L4, C5, WL7
Enlarged Thyroid	G1, M2, L4, C5	Kidney Infection or Stones	G1, M2, L4	Irregular Cycle	G1, CE3, L4, C5, WL7
Eye Pain	G1, M2, L4, C5	Tumors	G1, M2, L4 & * (WL7) or (ML8)	Lumps in Breasts	G1, CE3, L4, C5, WL7
Gum Trouble	G1, M2, L4, C5	**FECAL MATTER (Texture, Shape, Condition)**		Menopausal Symptoms	G1, CE3, L4, C5, WL7
Hay fever	G1, M2, L4, C5, B6	Dark brown	G1, M2, CE3, L4	Painful Menstruation	G1, CE3, L4, C5, WL7
Hoarseness	G1, M2, L4, C5, B6	Short in Shape/Size	G1, M2, CE3, L4	Tumors	G1, CE3, L4, C5, WL7
Gum Trouble	G1, M2, L4, C5			Menopausal Symptoms	G1, CE3, L4, C5, WL7

CIRCLES OF WELLNESS

Wellness Issue	Product Usage	Wellness Issue	Product Usage	Wellness Issue	Product Usage
Nose bleeds	G1, M2, L4, C5, B6			Vaginal Itch	G1, CE3, L4, C5, WL7
Sinus infection	G1, M2, L4, C5, B6			Hysterectomy	G1, M2, C5
Sore Throat	G1, M2, L4, C5, B6			If Miscarriage? How many? ___	G1, L4, C5, WL7
Tonsillitis	G1, M2, L4, C5, B6				

CODES: Green Life - G1 /Master Herbal – M2 /Colon Ease – CE3 /Laxative – L4 / Clay - CE5/ Breath of Life - B6 / Woman's Life - WL7/ Man's Life – ML8

*NOTE:

(WL7) or (ML8) When both listed – women use (WL7); men use (ML8)

NOTE:

For addressing all of these dis-eases setting up your home is paramount for securing your wellness. Refer to these three wellness home charts: (1) Nutrition Kitchen/ (2) 8 Pyramids of Wellness / (3) Hydro-therapy Bathroom

Disclaimer: this chart offers wellness suggestions. it is not intended to prescribe. Please consult your medical physician regarding your health.

(EMPOWERMENT)

12 EMPOWERMENT WHEEL CIRCLES

Each of the following Wellness Empowerment Circle Wheels focuses on a particular health challenge. Each health challenge is addressed by offering elemental recommendations through the use of herbs, dietary suggestions, heat treatments, hydrotherapy, flower essences and breath exercises that aid the body, mind, and spirit to rotate from a counter-clockwise dis-eased state to a clockwise vibrant healthy state of being.

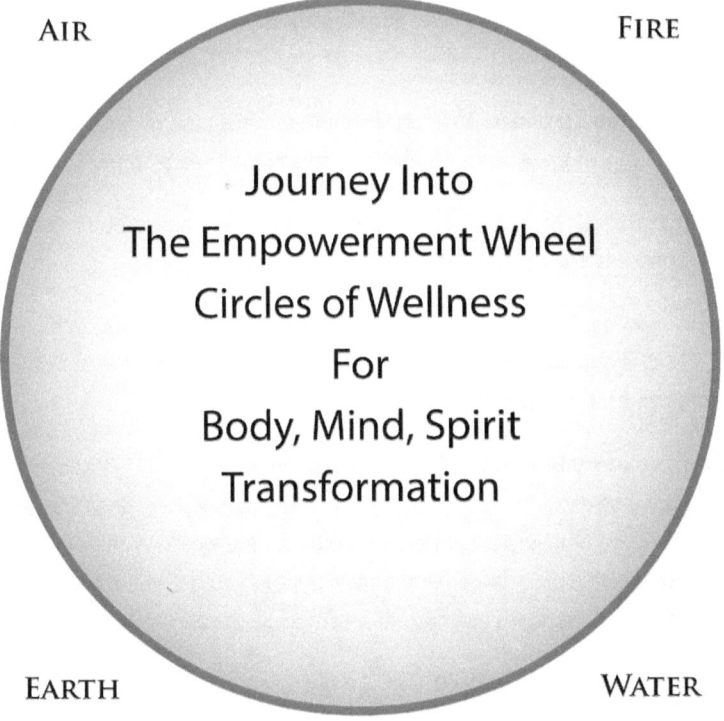

Blood and Circulatory Wellness Empowerment Guide

For High Blood Pressure Prevention

High blood pressure challenge: This occurs when as the heart pumps blood through the arteries, the blood presses against the walls of the blood vessels and the pressure is abnormally high. One may have primary blood pressure that shows up as only high blood pressure. The second form of pressure is called secondary high blood pressure, a result of obesity, stress, cigarette smoking, high sodium intake, coffee, and drug abuse. High blood pressure indicates that the walls on the arteries are filled with plaque.

Other related diseases: Blood Clots, Heart Attacks, Strokes, Headaches, Heart Failure, Kidney Failure, Excessive Sweating, Shortness of Breath, Dizziness, Water Retention

African American Statistics: 35% of African Americans have hypertension, which accounts for 20% of the African American deaths in the United States.

American Statistics: More than 60 million Americans have high blood pressure. 53% of Americans age 65-74 have high blood pressure

Global: Worldwide, high blood pressure is estimated to cause 7.1 million deaths, about 13% of the global fatality total. High blood pressure causes five million premature deaths a year worldwide

Blood & Circulatory Breath work: Breathe in a circular motion 20-40 times. Visualize your inhale as a circle of light coming into your body and exhale as you complete the circle and your breath expands out into the world. With each breath, your circle of light becomes larger and more vibrant as you become more and more relaxed. Cleanse your arteries in a circular breath through your body for 20-40 rounds

Blood & Circulatory Affirmation: My life is providing me with everything that I need and I am giving to life everything that life requires of me in a circular motion.

(EMPOWERMENT)

– 1 –
BLOOD AND CIRCULATORY WELLNESS EMPOWERMENT CIRCLE WHEEL FOR HIGH BLOOD PRESSURE PREVENTION

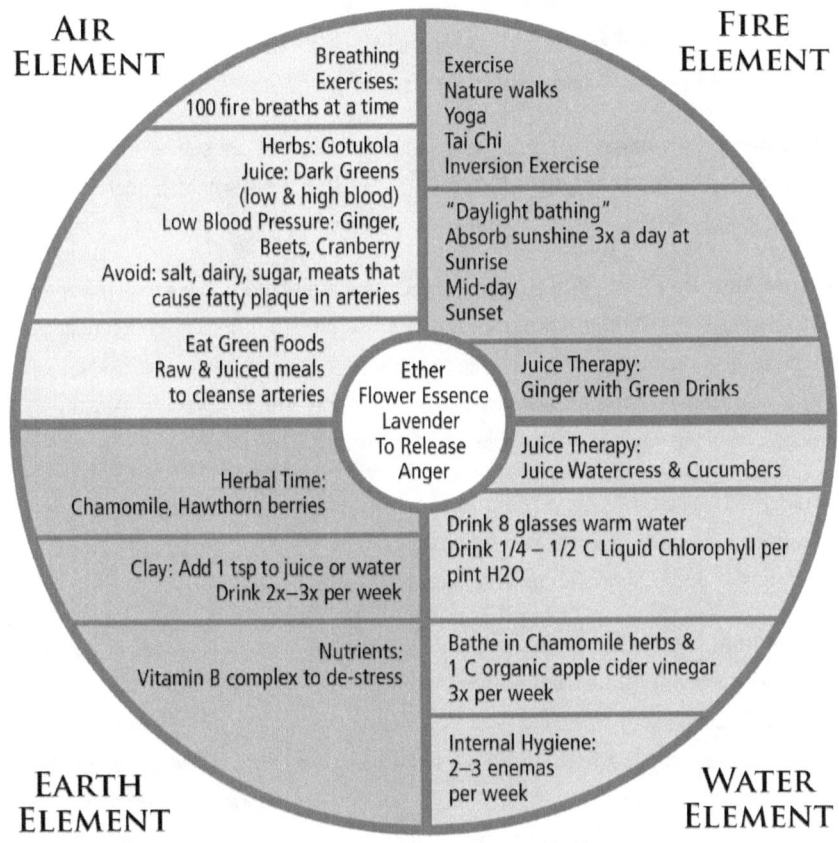

AIR ELEMENT
- Breathing Exercises: 100 fire breaths at a time
- Herbs: Gotukola
- Juice: Dark Greens (low & high blood)
- Low Blood Pressure: Ginger, Beets, Cranberry
- Avoid: salt, dairy, sugar, meats that cause fatty plaque in arteries

FIRE ELEMENT
- Exercise
- Nature walks
- Yoga
- Tai Chi
- Inversion Exercise
- "Daylight bathing" Absorb sunshine 3x a day at Sunrise Mid-day Sunset
- Juice Therapy: Ginger with Green Drinks
- Juice Therapy: Juice Watercress & Cucumbers

Ether
Flower Essence Lavender To Release Anger

EARTH ELEMENT
- Eat Green Foods Raw & Juiced meals to cleanse arteries
- Herbal Time: Chamomile, Hawthorn berries
- Clay: Add 1 tsp to juice or water Drink 2x–3x per week
- Nutrients: Vitamin B complex to de-stress

WATER ELEMENT
- Drink 8 glasses warm water Drink 1/4 – 1/2 C Liquid Chlorophyll per pint H2O
- Bathe in Chamomile herbs & 1 C organic apple cider vinegar 3x per week
- Internal Hygiene: 2–3 enemas per week

Disclaimer: The information in this chart offers wellness recommendations and suggestions, and is not intended to diagnose or prescribe. Please consult with your medical physician regarding your health.

Bone and Joint Wellness Empowerment Guide
For Arthritis Prevention

Bone Deterioration Challenge: Bone loss, also known as osteoporosis, is brought on by specific diseases and/or long-term use of certain medications. Bone is living tissue in a constant cycle of loss and replacement within the body. When osteoporosis occurs, new bone replacement is not keeping up with old bone loss. The old, weakened bones are at risk of fracture, particularly the hips, wrists and spine. Foods rich in calcium, vitamin D and other nutrients are important for bone wellness.

Other related dis-eases: Arthritis, Back Pain, Disorders of Connective Tissue, need for Hip and/or Knee Replacement, Osteoarthritis, Rheumatoid Arthritis, Scoliosis Arthritis, Swollen Joints. Also, Oral bone loss and Tooth decay and loss.

African American Statistics: African American women tend to have higher bone mineral density (BMD) than Caucasian American women, but are still at significant risk of developing osteoporosis. The misconception that bone loss is a problem only for Caucasian American women delays prevention and treatment by African American women who do not believe they are at risk for the disease.

American Statistics: Osteoporosis affects millions of Americans. Many with osteoporosis are at high risk of suffering one or more fractures, which can present challenges to both physical and mental wellness.

Bone & Joint Breath Work: Meditate and breathe deeply as you fill your bones with hope and stamina. Sit on a comfortable chair. Align your head with your shoulders and your feet with your hips. Place your feet flat on the floor and your hands in your lap with palms facing upward. Align your mind with your heart, and your heart with your body. Inhale through your nostrils as you expand your lungs and abdomen. Exhale from your nostrils as you contract your abdomen and relax your lungs. Perform this breathing of 20 - 100 lotus fire breaths 2 - 3 times a day. If you consciously practice the full body breath, in time it will become your norm. With each breath, your body will be more and more enlivened. Over a season, increase to 1000 lotus fire breaths daily. Perform 250 lotus fire breaths at: sunrise, midday, sunset, before bed.

Bone & Joint Affirmation: I come into being from unformed matter. Make me always prosperous. Triumphantly gather my bones & collect my limbs.

(EMPOWERMENT)

– 2 –

BONE AND JOINT WELLNESS EMPOWERMENT CIRCLE WHEEL FOR ARTHRITIS PREVENTION

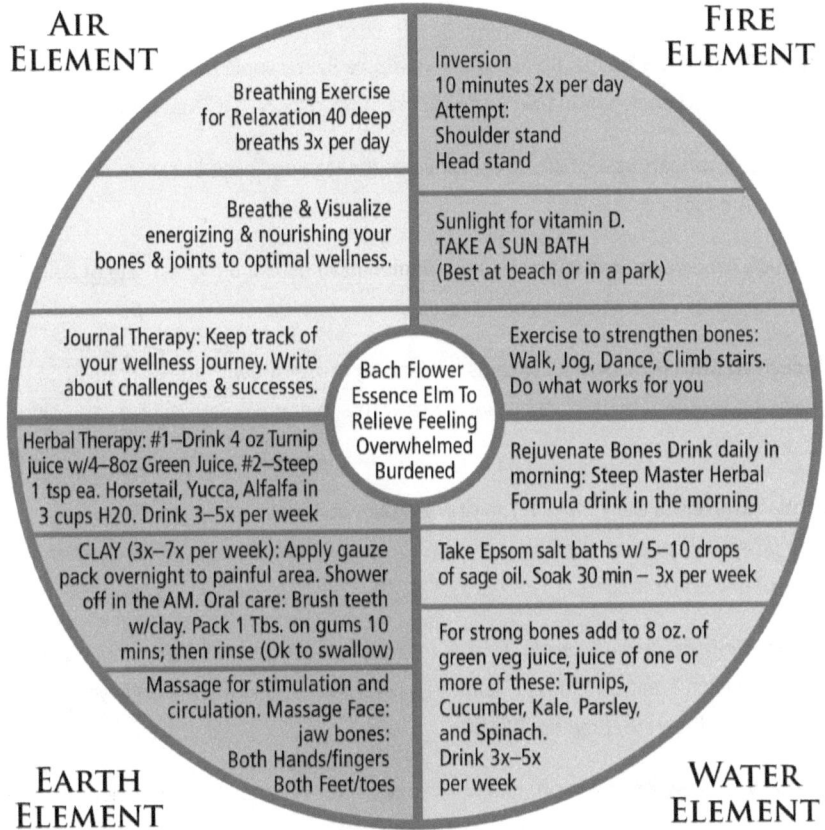

AIR ELEMENT

- Breathing Exercise for Relaxation 40 deep breaths 3x per day
- Breathe & Visualize energizing & nourishing your bones & joints to optimal wellness.

FIRE ELEMENT

- Inversion 10 minutes 2x per day Attempt: Shoulder stand Head stand
- Sunlight for vitamin D. TAKE A SUN BATH (Best at beach or in a park)

EARTH ELEMENT

- Journal Therapy: Keep track of your wellness journey. Write about challenges & successes.
- Herbal Therapy: #1—Drink 4 oz Turnip juice w/4–8oz Green Juice. #2—Steep 1 tsp ea. Horsetail, Yucca, Alfalfa in 3 cups H20. Drink 3–5x per week
- CLAY (3x–7x per week): Apply gauze pack overnight to painful area. Shower off in the AM. Oral care: Brush teeth w/clay. Pack 1 Tbs. on gums 10 mins; then rinse (Ok to swallow)
- Massage for stimulation and circulation. Massage Face: jaw bones: Both Hands/fingers Both Feet/toes

WATER ELEMENT

- Exercise to strengthen bones: Walk, Jog, Dance, Climb stairs. Do what works for you
- Rejuvenate Bones Drink daily in morning: Steep Master Herbal Formula drink in the morning
- Take Epsom salt baths w/ 5–10 drops of sage oil. Soak 30 min – 3x per week
- For strong bones add to 8 oz. of green veg juice, juice of one or more of these: Turnips, Cucumber, Kale, Parsley, and Spinach. Drink 3x–5x per week

Center: Bach Flower Essence Elm To Relieve Feeling Overwhelmed Burdened

Disclaimer: The information in this chart offers wellness recommendations and suggestions, and is not intended to diagnose or prescribe. Please consult with your medical physician regarding your health.

Breast Wellness Empowerment Guide
For Cancer Prevention

Breast Cancer Challenge: A lump forms in the breast that is cancerous within the lobes, milk ducts, and fatty tissues of the breast. Breast cancer is primarily due to high levels of Estrogen in the blood stream. Estrogen promotes cellular growth in the tissues of the breast

Other Related Dis-eases: Breast Swelling, Nipple Pain, Nipple Discharge, Red Scaling Or Thickening Of The Skin And Nipple, Inward Curve Of The Nipple

African American Statistics: Breast cancer is the leading cause of cancer death for African American women

Spanish American Statistics: Hispanic women have the third highest rate of deaths from breast cancer amongst all other races.

American Statistics: Breast cancer is the leading cause of death for women 40-55 years of age. The rate of incidence increases with age and women 75 years and older are at highest risk

Global Statistics: More than 1.1 million women worldwide are newly diagnosed with breast cancer annually. This represents about 10% of all new cancer cases and 23% of all female cancers

Breast Wellness Breath work: Breathe into your breast, your seat of nurturing and love, with each breath. Increase a self nurturing spirit. Expand and magnify your inner love with each breath. Breathe 40-100x

Breast Wellness Affirmation: I mentally and physically caress the expression of love that is emanating from the heart of my breast.

(EMPOWERMENT)

– 3 –

BREAST WELLNESS EMPOWERMENT CIRCLE WHEEL FOR CANCER PREVENTION

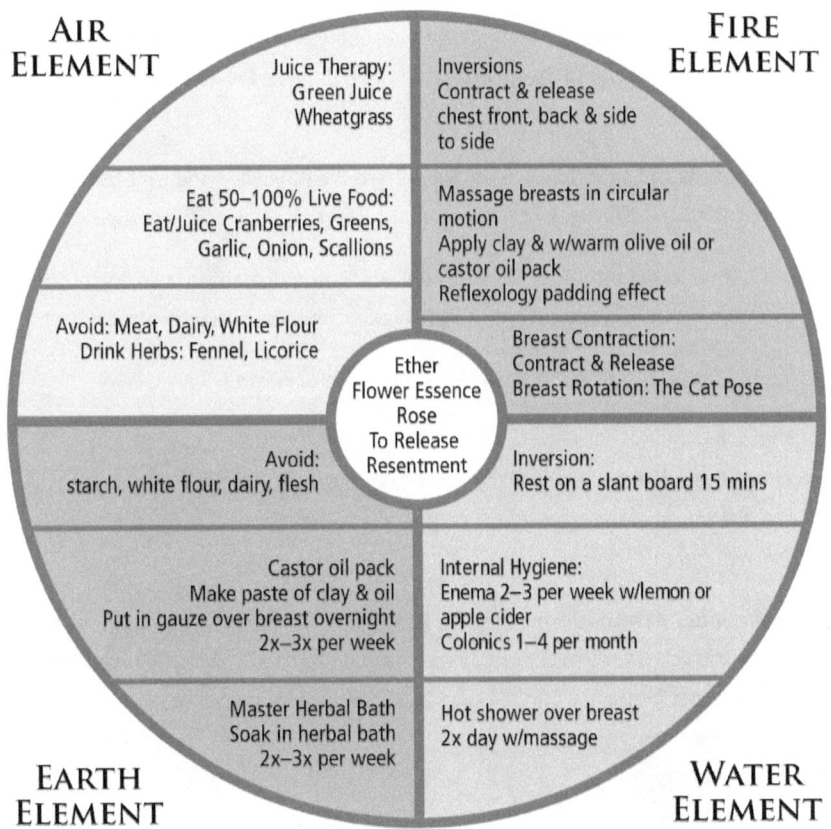

Disclaimer: The information in this chart offers wellness recommendations and suggestions, and is not intended to diagnose or prescribe. Please consult with your medical physician regarding your health.

Colon Wellness Empowerment Guide
For Constipation Prevention

Constipation Challenge: This occurs when the stool is hard and impacted in the colon, and it cannot easily move through the colon. Dr. Robert Wood teaches that 80-90% of disease begins from waste impacted in the colon walls.

Other Related Dis-eases: Gas, Indigestion, Abdominal Bloating, Prolapsed Colon, Prolapsed Womb, Prolapsed Bladder, Sluggishness, Blocked Prostate, Mood Swings, Stress

African American Statistics: Black women have the highest incidence of and mortality from colon and rectal cancer than any other ethnic or racial group

Spanish American Statistics: Survival rates after being diagnosed with colon cancer are lower for Hispanics, due to lack of Self-Health care, and quality treatment

American: Colon cancer is the second leading cause of death from cancer in the United States.

Colon Wellness Breath work: Allow your inner breath to become light and even. Breathe the breath of life through your colon as you cleanse and purge the fecal impaction out with each breath

Colon Wellness Affirmation: I affirm to keep my colon cleansed from toxic heavy thoughts which cause me to consume heavy toxic foods. I will lift my mind and spirit up to the highest frequency that my colon will be free of toxicity.

(EMPOWERMENT)

– 4 –

COLON WELLNESS EMPOWERMENT CIRCLE WHEEL FOR CONSTIPATION PREVENTION

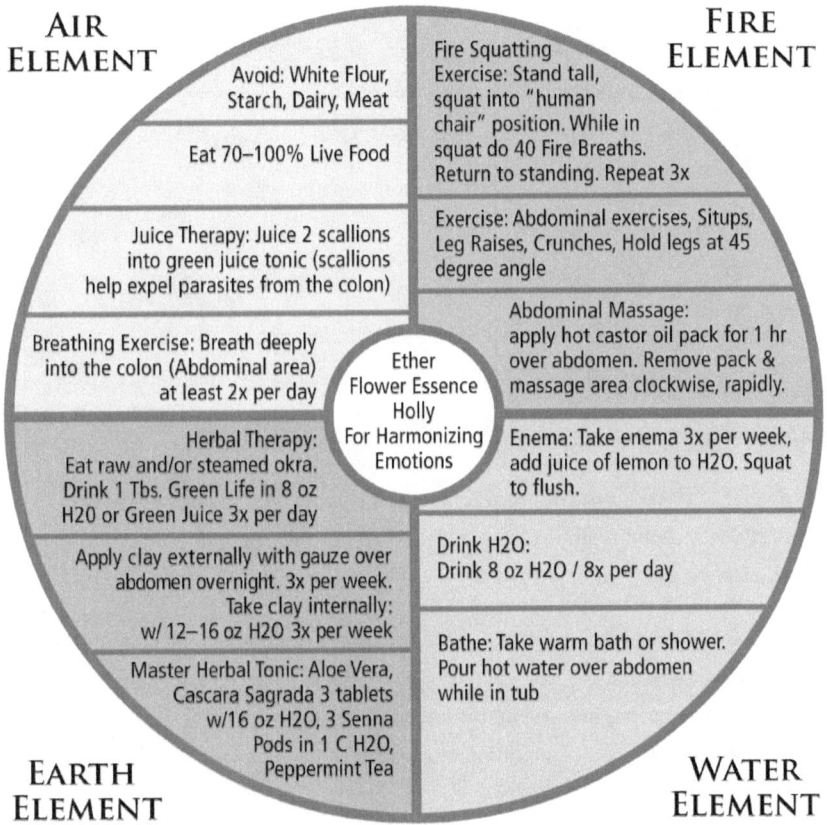

AIR ELEMENT

- Avoid: White Flour, Starch, Dairy, Meat
- Eat 70–100% Live Food
- Juice Therapy: Juice 2 scallions into green juice tonic (scallions help expel parasites from the colon)
- Breathing Exercise: Breath deeply into the colon (Abdominal area) at least 2x per day
- Herbal Therapy: Eat raw and/or steamed okra. Drink 1 Tbs. Green Life in 8 oz H2O or Green Juice 3x per day

FIRE ELEMENT

- Fire Squatting Exercise: Stand tall, squat into "human chair" position. While in squat do 40 Fire Breaths. Return to standing. Repeat 3x
- Exercise: Abdominal exercises, Situps, Leg Raises, Crunches, Hold legs at 45 degree angle
- Abdominal Massage: apply hot castor oil pack for 1 hr over abdomen. Remove pack & massage area clockwise, rapidly.
- Enema: Take enema 3x per week, add juice of lemon to H2O. Squat to flush.

Ether Flower Essence Holly For Harmonizing Emotions

EARTH ELEMENT

- Apply clay externally with gauze over abdomen overnight. 3x per week. Take clay internally: w/ 12–16 oz H2O 3x per week
- Master Herbal Tonic: Aloe Vera, Cascara Sagrada 3 tablets w/16 oz H2O, 3 Senna Pods in 1 C H2O, Peppermint Tea

WATER ELEMENT

- Drink H2O: Drink 8 oz H2O / 8x per day
- Bathe: Take warm bath or shower. Pour hot water over abdomen while in tub

Disclaimer: The information in this chart offers wellness recommendations and suggestions, and is not intended to diagnose or prescribe. Please consult with your medical physician regarding your health.

Emotional Wellness Empowerment Guide
For Stress Prevention

Obesity Challenge: When one is 20% over the body fat of their normal weight for their age, gender, height and build.

Other Related Dis-ease: Stress, Anxiety, Mood Swings, Obesity, Depression, Bi-polar conditions

African American Statistics: More than half of all African Americans are anticipated to use public insurance to pay for inpatient emotional health treatment, compared to 34% of Caucasians.

American Statistics: more than 25 million Americans have emotional stress as the cause of their Physical ailments

Global Statistics: Depression is one of the most common conditions in young people and increases during adolescence

Emotional Balancing: I release all stress from my life.

Emotional Wellness Breathe work: I breathe into my heart center a breath of lightness. With each breath I release the heaviness of this world (Breathe 20 breaths before each meal.)

Emotional Wellness Affirmation: I am emotionally centered and in divine order. I can handle with ease and grace all challenges. For all challenges are opportunities for me to grow, to expand, and to improve my life. I am filled with love and gratitude. All I need is with is within me. I am emotionally balanced.

(EMPOWERMENT)

– 5 –
EMOTIONAL WELLNESS EMPOWERMENT CIRCLE WHEEL FOR STRESS PREVENTION

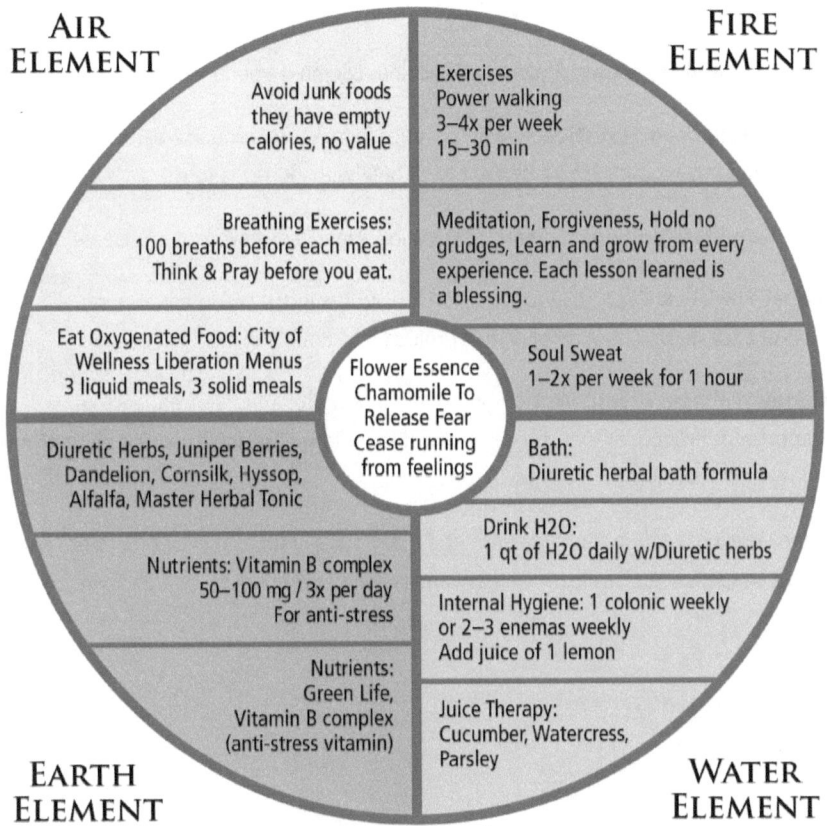

AIR ELEMENT
- Avoid Junk foods they have empty calories, no value
- Breathing Exercises: 100 breaths before each meal. Think & Pray before you eat.
- Eat Oxygenated Food: City of Wellness Liberation Menus 3 liquid meals, 3 solid meals
- Diuretic Herbs, Juniper Berries, Dandelion, Cornsilk, Hyssop, Alfalfa, Master Herbal Tonic

FIRE ELEMENT
- Exercises Power walking 3–4x per week 15–30 min
- Meditation, Forgiveness, Hold no grudges, Learn and grow from every experience. Each lesson learned is a blessing.
- Soul Sweat 1–2x per week for 1 hour
- Bath: Diuretic herbal bath formula

EARTH ELEMENT
- Nutrients: Vitamin B complex 50–100 mg / 3x per day For anti-stress
- Nutrients: Green Life, Vitamin B complex (anti-stress vitamin)

WATER ELEMENT
- Drink H2O: 1 qt of H2O daily w/Diuretic herbs
- Internal Hygiene: 1 colonic weekly or 2–3 enemas weekly Add juice of 1 lemon
- Juice Therapy: Cucumber, Watercress, Parsley

Center: Flower Essence Chamomile To Release Fear Cease running from feelings

Disclaimer: The information in this chart offers wellness recommendations and suggestions, and is not intended to diagnose or prescribe. Please consult with your medical physician regarding your health.

KIDNEY WELLNESS EMPOWERMENT GUIDE
For Edema and Kidney Failure Prevention

Kidney Challenge: Kidneys remove our waste from the body to regulate fluid balance in the body. Urine (waste) production wanes because when the kidneys are unable to properly excrete salt and other wastes, which leads to the accumulation of toxic waste in the body.

Other Related Dis-eases: Protein in the Urine, Edema, Hypertension

African American Statistics: African Americans make up about 12 percent of the population but account for 32 percent of people with kidney failure

American Statistics: Approximately 20 million Americans have kidney disease

Global Statistics: Today, over one million individuals in the world are alive on maintenance dialysis, a number that is projected to double in the next decade.

Kidney Wellness Breath Work: I breathe in a new life, a higher frequency of supportive fulfilling relations. I breathe out disappointments and hurt. The spirit of my Kidney is restored

Kidney Wellness Affirmation: I release and drain out all hurt and disappointment from my past experiences. I welcome in new and fulfilling experiences with all my relations

(Empowerment)

– 6 –

Kidney Wellness
Empowerment Circle Wheel
For Edema and Kidney Failure Prevention

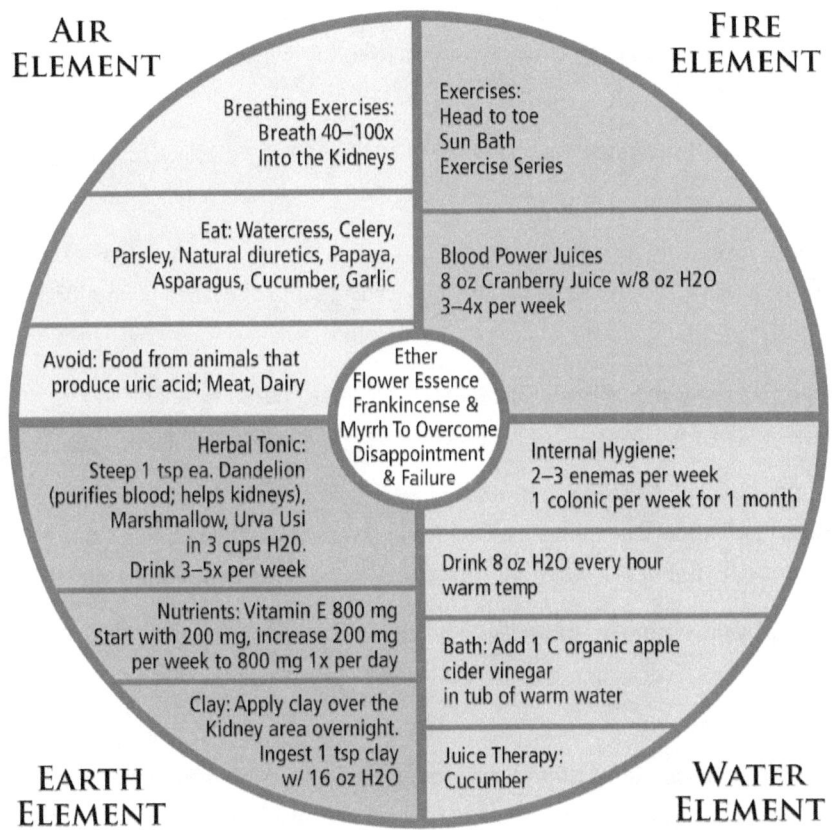

AIR ELEMENT
- Breathing Exercises: Breath 40–100x Into the Kidneys
- Eat: Watercress, Celery, Parsley, Natural diuretics, Papaya, Asparagus, Cucumber, Garlic
- Avoid: Food from animals that produce uric acid; Meat, Dairy

FIRE ELEMENT
- Exercises: Head to toe Sun Bath Exercise Series
- Blood Power Juices 8 oz Cranberry Juice w/8 oz H2O 3–4x per week

Ether
Flower Essence Frankincense & Myrrh To Overcome Disappointment & Failure

EARTH ELEMENT
- Herbal Tonic: Steep 1 tsp ea. Dandelion (purifies blood; helps kidneys), Marshmallow, Urva Usi in 3 cups H2O. Drink 3–5x per week
- Nutrients: Vitamin E 800 mg Start with 200 mg, increase 200 mg per week to 800 mg 1x per day
- Clay: Apply clay over the Kidney area overnight. Ingest 1 tsp clay w/ 16 oz H2O

WATER ELEMENT
- Internal Hygiene: 2–3 enemas per week 1 colonic per week for 1 month
- Drink 8 oz H2O every hour warm temp
- Bath: Add 1 C organic apple cider vinegar in tub of warm water
- Juice Therapy: Cucumber

Herbal Kidney Circle Tonic available from The Queen Afua Wellness Center

Disclaimer: The information in this chart offers wellness recommendations and suggestions, and is not intended to diagnose or prescribe. Please consult with your medical physician regarding your health.

Mental Wellness Empowerment Guide
For Depression and Alzheimer's' Prevention

Depression Challenge: Depression affects the entire body, the thoughts, nerves, and emotions. Depression is a psychological imbalance that has a physical impact on the anatomy particularly the nervous system. There are 2 types of depression. One is uni-polar which occurs a few times in the course of one's lifetime. The second type of depression is bi-polar, which alternates between depression and manic chronic depression

Other Related Dis-eases: Fatigue, Depression, Headaches, Irritability, Anxiety, Bi-polar conditions

African American Statistics: in 2004, 2,019 African Americans completed suicide, and was recently ranked as the third leading cause of death among African Americans

Spanish American Statistics: One study found in their health survey, over 26% of their samples were depressed, and more than 20% of the cases related to physical health

Global Statistics: Self-inflicted injuries, due to mental illness, represented 1.8% of the global burden of disease in 1998 and are expected to increase to 2.4%t in 2020

Mental Wellness Breath Work: Perform a sweeping breath through my feet, spine, head, and heart, back down into my feet. I breathe a circle of love that surrounds my entire being.

Anti-stress Relaxation Affirmation: Today I send sun rays of serenity and inner peace through the soles of my feet to my spine, to my head and down into my heart

(EMPOWERMENT)

– 7 –

MENTAL WELLNESS
EMPOWERMENT CIRCLE WHEEL
FOR DEPRESSION AND ALZHEIMER'S' PREVENTION

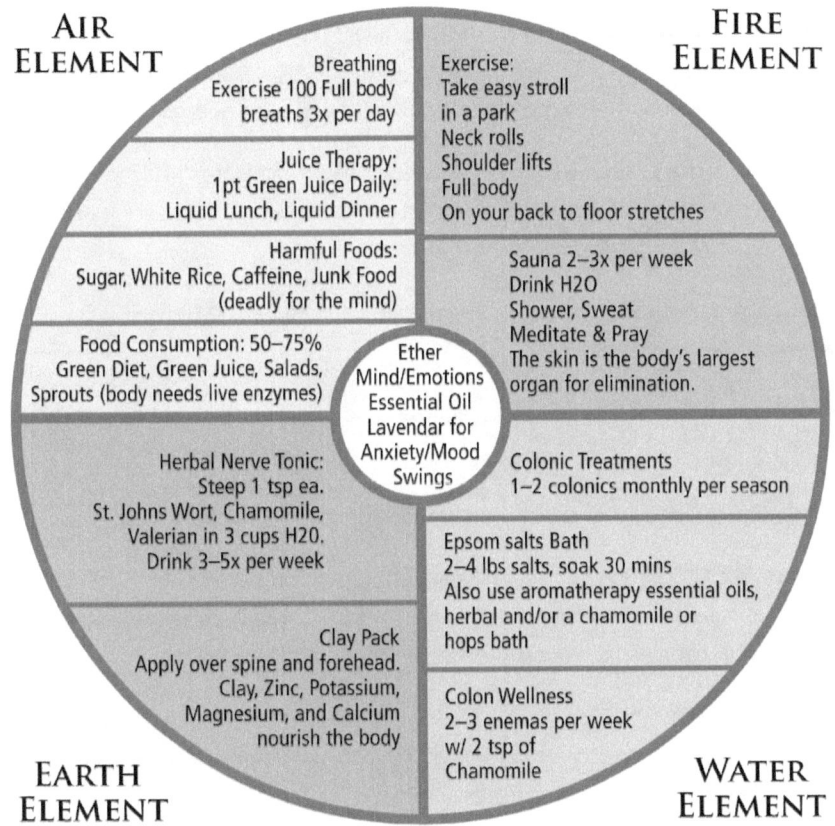

Herbal Mental Wellness Circle Tonic available from The Queen Afua Wellness Center

Disclaimer: The information in this chart offers wellness recommendations and suggestions, and is not intended to diagnose or prescribe. Please consult with your medical physician regarding your health.

PANCREATIC WELLNESS EMPOWERMENT GUIDE
For Diabetes Prevention

Diabetes Challenge: This occurs when the body is unable to regulate glucose. Glucose is the fuel used by cells to produce energy and insulin, the hormone that helps glucose enter the cells.

Other Related Dis-eases: Fatigue, Thirst, Frequent Urination, Blood Sugar Concerns that can cause Dizziness, Obesity, Diabetically damaged Nerves and Blood Vessels throughout the body, which may cause neuropathy and eye dis-ease.

African American Statistics: African Americans have the highest incidence of pancreatic cancer of any ethnic group worldwide. Whether this difference is due to diet or environmental factors remains unclear.

Spanish American Statistics: 12,320 Hispanic men and 11,000 Hispanic women were expected to die from Cancer on 2006.

American Statistics: Prevalence of Diagnosed and Undiagnosed Diabetes in the United States, All Ages, 2007.

Total: 23.6 million people—7.8 percent of the population—have diabetes.

Diagnosed: 17.9 million people. Undiagnosed: 5.7 million people. About 186,300 people younger than 20 years have diabetes—type 1 or type 2. This represents 0.2 percent of all people in this age group.

Global Statistics: Although the U.S. is expected to experience a far more rapid increase in diabetes rates, the study suggests the greatest relative increases will be in the Middle East, sub-Saharan Africa, and India.

Pancreatic Wellness Breath work: Breathe joy and kindness, love and sweetness into your blood stream, your pancreas and your kidneys. I am fulfilled.

Pancreatic Wellness Affirmation: Thoughts of kindness and sweetness permeates my bloodstream, my Pancreas, and my Kidneys, undammed, I flow in the spirit of joy

(EMPOWERMENT)

– 8 –

PANCREATIC WELLNESS EMPOWERMENT CIRCLE WHEEL FOR DIABETES PREVENTION

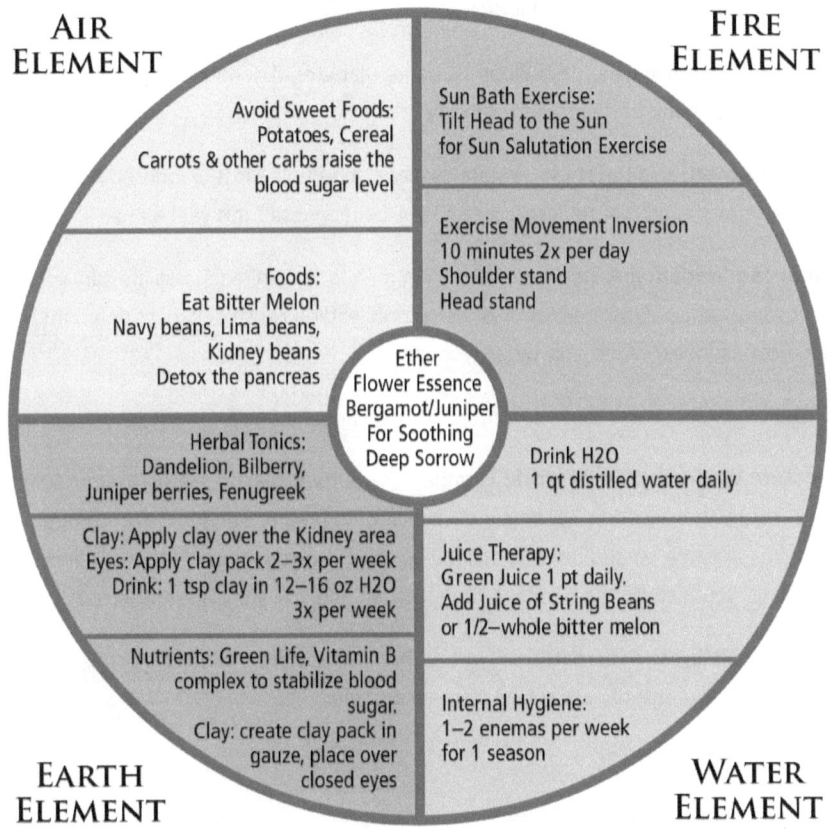

Herbal Diabetic Circle Tonic available from The Queen Afua Wellness Center

Disclaimer: The information in this chart offers wellness recommendations and suggestions, and is not intended to diagnose or prescribe. Please consult with your medical physician regarding your health.

Prostate Wellness Empowerment Guide
For Impotency Prevention

Impotency: Is an erectile dysfunction which occurs when a man is unable to achieve or maintain an erection for sexual intercourse. Impotency is due to lack of brain blood vessels stimulating nerve functioning and hormonal action. Any one of these malfunctions can lead to vascular disease.

Other related diseases: High Blood Pressure, Diabetes, Arteriosclerosis, Edema in legs, Poor Circulation, Depression, Anxiety

African American Statistics: Prostate cancer is the single most diagnosed non-skin cancer among African Americans: 30,870 will be diagnosed this year alone.

American Statistics: A little over 1.8 million men in the United States are survivors of prostate cancer. Prostate cancer is the second leading cause of cancer death in American men, exceeded only by lung cancer

Global: Prostate cancer ranks second after lung cancer in male cancer deaths

Prostate Wellness Breath work: Breathe into your vascular circulatory system from your feet to your prostate. Breathe a deep cleansing breath; out and down through your legs. Breathe up and down through your legs into your prostate 40-100 times. Each time you breathe the breath is strengthened and you are left empowered.

Prostate Wellness Affirmations: I affirm that my prostate is vibrant, electric, rejuvenated and nutritionally sound. I am empowered.

(EMPOWERMENT)

– 9 –

PROSTATE WELLNESS EMPOWERMENT CIRCLE WHEEL FOR IMPOTENCY PREVENTION

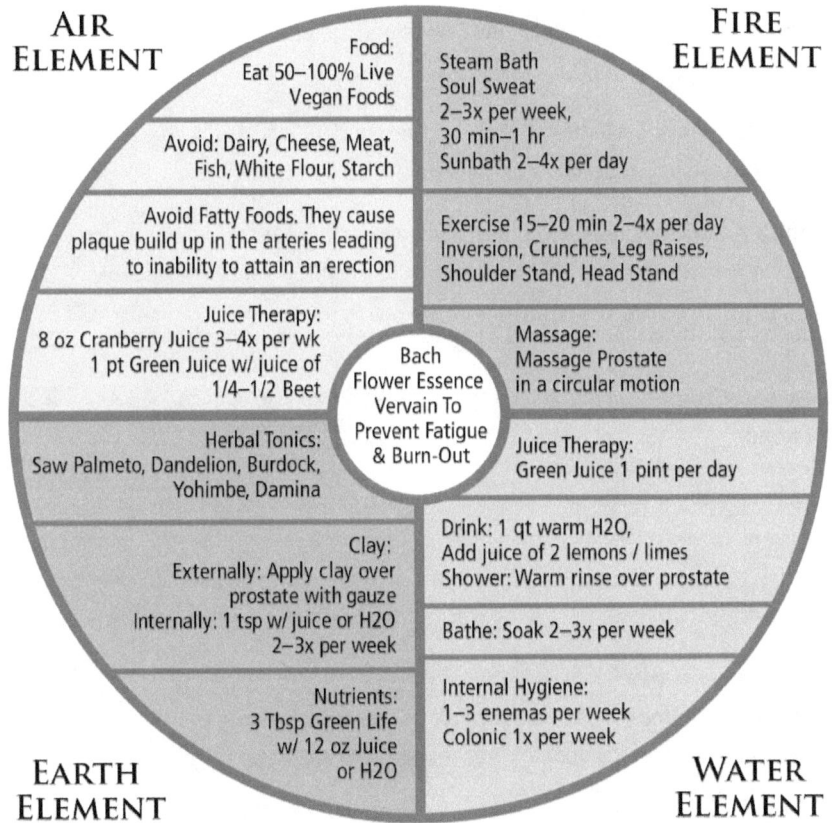

AIR ELEMENT

Food: Eat 50–100% Live Vegan Foods

Avoid: Dairy, Cheese, Meat, Fish, White Flour, Starch

Avoid Fatty Foods. They cause plaque build up in the arteries leading to inability to attain an erection

Juice Therapy: 8 oz Cranberry Juice 3–4x per wk 1 pt Green Juice w/ juice of 1/4–1/2 Beet

Herbal Tonics: Saw Palmeto, Dandelion, Burdock, Yohimbe, Damina

FIRE ELEMENT

Steam Bath Soul Sweat 2–3x per week, 30 min–1 hr Sunbath 2–4x per day

Exercise 15–20 min 2–4x per day Inversion, Crunches, Leg Raises, Shoulder Stand, Head Stand

Massage: Massage Prostate in a circular motion

Juice Therapy: Green Juice 1 pint per day

Bach Flower Essence Vervain To Prevent Fatigue & Burn-Out

Clay: Externally: Apply clay over prostate with gauze Internally: 1 tsp w/ juice or H2O 2–3x per week

Nutrients: 3 Tbsp Green Life w/ 12 oz Juice or H2O

EARTH ELEMENT

Drink: 1 qt warm H2O, Add juice of 2 lemons / limes Shower: Warm rinse over prostate

Bathe: Soak 2–3x per week

Internal Hygiene: 1–3 enemas per week Colonic 1x per week

WATER ELEMENT

Heal Thyself Mens Life Prostate Wellness Tonic available from The Queen Afua Wellness Center

Disclaimer: The information in this chart offers wellness recommendations and suggestions, and is not intended to diagnose or prescribe. Please consult with your medical physician regarding your health.

Respiratory Wellness Empowerment Guide
For Asthma Prevention

Asthmatic Challenge: is a respiratory dis-ease that is due to obstruction in the lungs and constriction of the air passages in the chest. Symptoms: tightness in the chest and shortness of breath, causing other related dis-eases.

Other related dis-eases: Colds, Hay Fever, Snoring, Bronchitis, Wheezing, Hoarseness

African American Statistics: Asthma prevalence is 39% higher in African Americans than in Caucasian Americans.

Spanish American Statistics: In the Childhood Asthma Project funded at the UT Health Science Center, of the 145 subjects enrolled, 115(79%) were Hispanic

American Statistics: Asthma and allergies strike 1 out of 4 Americans

Global Statistics: Australia has the third highest prevalence of childhood Asthma in the world

Respiratory Wellness Breath Work: I center my body, mind, spirit and lungs as I breathe deep into my lungs I expand my ribcage as I release my breath. I relax from all tension deeper and deeper with each breath. I release mental emotional and physical pressure from my lungs. As I count from 10-0 my lungs become more at ease.

Respiratory Wellness Affirmation: Today I release constriction and confusion from my life as I breathe in freedom and expansion. With each breath I take, my lungs are restored to balance and harmony.

(EMPOWERMENT)

– 10 –
Respiratory Wellness Empowerment Circle Wheel For Asthma Prevention

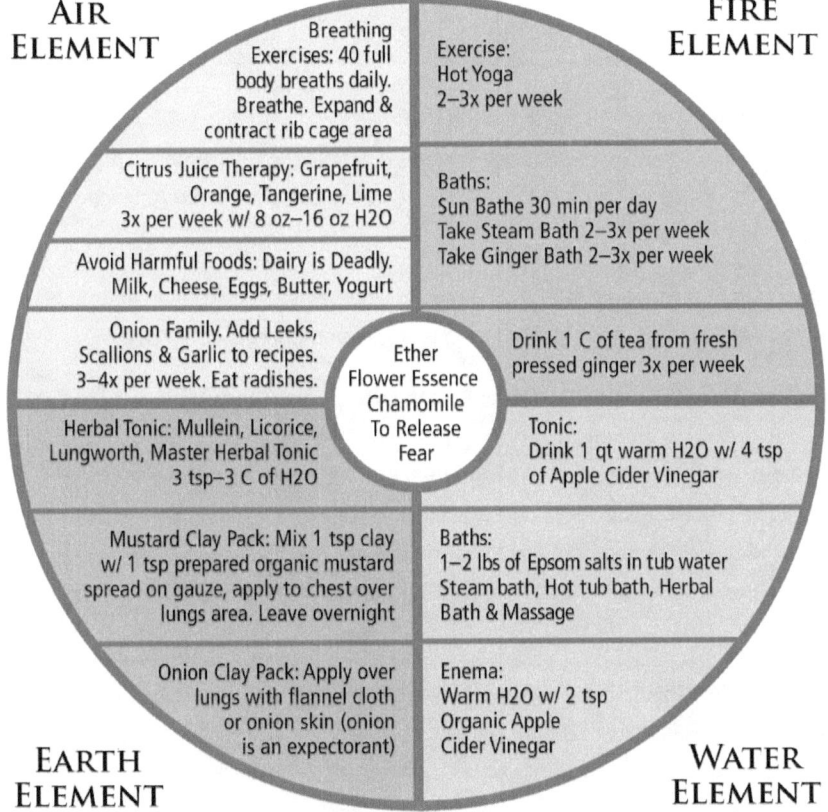

AIR ELEMENT
- Breathing Exercises: 40 full body breaths daily. Breathe. Expand & contract rib cage area
- Citrus Juice Therapy: Grapefruit, Orange, Tangerine, Lime 3x per week w/ 8 oz–16 oz H2O
- Avoid Harmful Foods: Dairy is Deadly. Milk, Cheese, Eggs, Butter, Yogurt
- Onion Family. Add Leeks, Scallions & Garlic to recipes. 3–4x per week. Eat radishes.
- Herbal Tonic: Mullein, Licorice, Lungwort, Master Herbal Tonic 3 tsp–3 C of H2O

FIRE ELEMENT
- Exercise: Hot Yoga 2–3x per week
- Baths: Sun Bathe 30 min per day Take Steam Bath 2–3x per week Take Ginger Bath 2–3x per week
- Drink 1 C of tea from fresh pressed ginger 3x per week
- Tonic: Drink 1 qt warm H2O w/ 4 tsp of Apple Cider Vinegar

Ether Flower Essence Chamomile To Release Fear

EARTH ELEMENT
- Mustard Clay Pack: Mix 1 tsp clay w/ 1 tsp prepared organic mustard spread on gauze, apply to chest over lungs area. Leave overnight
- Onion Clay Pack: Apply over lungs with flannel cloth or onion skin (onion is an expectorant)

WATER ELEMENT
- Baths: 1–2 lbs of Epsom salts in tub water Steam bath, Hot tub bath, Herbal Bath & Massage
- Enema: Warm H2O w/ 2 tsp Organic Apple Cider Vinegar

Herbal Respiratory Circle Tonic available from The Queen Afua Wellness Center

Disclaimer: The information in this chart offers wellness recommendations and suggestions, and is not intended to diagnose or prescribe. Please consult with your medical physician regarding your health.

Vibrant and Youthful Skin Wellness Empowerment Guide

For a Eczema and Acne Prevention

Acne Challenge: is an imbalance on the skin which manifests as blackheads and pimples that erupt through the pores on the face. A boil is a skin infection, a pus pocket that itches and swells and is filled with mucus congestion.

Other related dis-eases: Psoriasis, Eczema, Acne, Black heads, Boils, Loss of hair.

African American Statistics: Historically psoriasis was assumed to be a rare condition among African Americans, occurring in about 0.7 percent of the population (as compared to the 2.2 to 2.6 percent prevalence in the American population at large).

American Statistics: An estimated fifteen million people in the United States alone exhibit symptoms of atopic dermatitis, the most common form of eczema.

Vibrant & Youthful Skin Wellness Breath Work: Sit in a comfortable chair or in the tub; relax and breathe. Inhale deep into your face and breathe into your chin and then out. Breathe into your cheeks and then out. As you relax, breathe into your eyes and your temples and breathe out. Breathe into your forehead and then breathe out all of the stress. Breathe from the center of the face and exhale the relaxed breath around the entire face in a circular flow. Continue to breathe serenity and wellness in and out.

Vibrant & Youthful Skin Wellness Affirmation: My entire body is breathing and circulating love and inner peace. "My face is of Ra". My face is of light. I am free of anger and resentment. My skin is vibrant, alive and healthy because peace flows from my heart.

(EMPOWERMENT)

– 11 –
Vibrant and Youthful Skin Wellness Empowerment Circle Wheel For Eczema and Acne Prevention

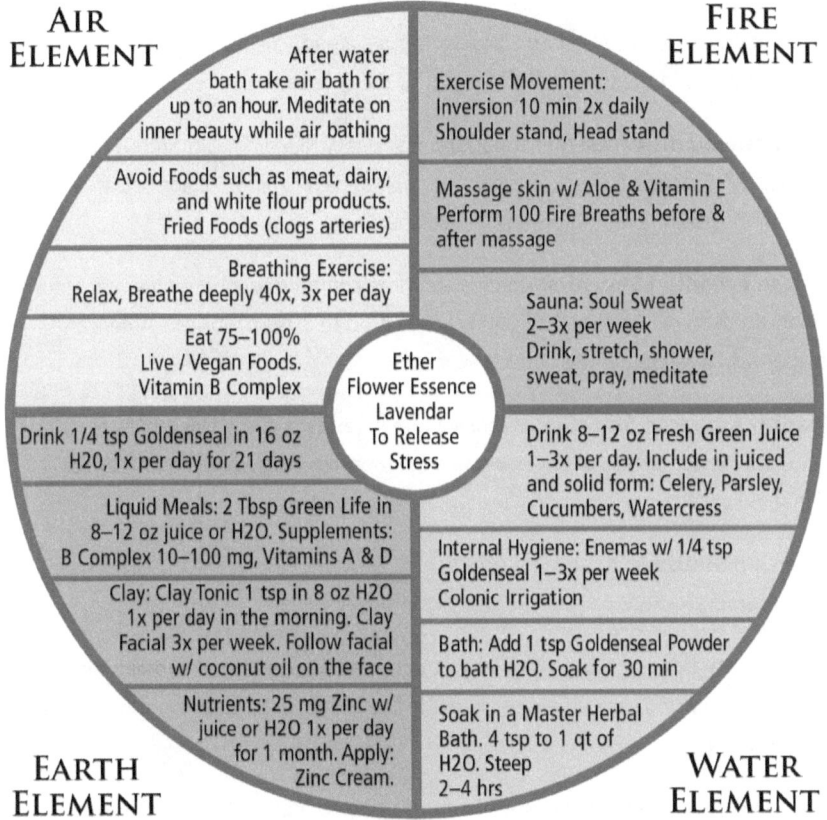

Air Element
- After water bath take air bath for up to an hour. Meditate on inner beauty while air bathing
- Avoid Foods such as meat, dairy, and white flour products. Fried Foods (clogs arteries)
- Breathing Exercise: Relax, Breathe deeply 40x, 3x per day

Fire Element
- Exercise Movement: Inversion 10 min 2x daily Shoulder stand, Head stand
- Massage skin w/ Aloe & Vitamin E Perform 100 Fire Breaths before & after massage
- Sauna: Soul Sweat 2–3x per week Drink, stretch, shower, sweat, pray, meditate

Earth Element
- Eat 75–100% Live / Vegan Foods. Vitamin B Complex
- Drink 1/4 tsp Goldenseal in 16 oz H2O, 1x per day for 21 days
- Liquid Meals: 2 Tbsp Green Life in 8–12 oz juice or H2O. Supplements: B Complex 10–100 mg, Vitamins A & D
- Clay: Clay Tonic 1 tsp in 8 oz H2O 1x per day in the morning. Clay Facial 3x per week. Follow facial w/ coconut oil on the face
- Nutrients: 25 mg Zinc w/ juice or H2O 1x per day for 1 month. Apply: Zinc Cream.

Water Element
- Drink 8–12 oz Fresh Green Juice 1–3x per day. Include in juiced and solid form: Celery, Parsley, Cucumbers, Watercress
- Internal Hygiene: Enemas w/ 1/4 tsp Goldenseal 1–3x per week Colonic Irrigation
- Bath: Add 1 tsp Goldenseal Powder to bath H2O. Soak for 30 min
- Soak in a Master Herbal Bath. 4 tsp to 1 qt of H2O. Steep 2–4 hrs

Ether Flower Essence Lavendar To Release Stress

Disclaimer: The information in this chart offers wellness recommendations and suggestions, and is not intended to diagnose or prescribe. Please consult with your medical physician regarding your health.

Womb Wellness Fibroid Free Empowerment Guide
For Fibroid Tumor Prevention

Fibroid Tumor Challenge: A benign growth that is on the walls of the uterus. Fibroid origins, often "misunderstood" by scientists, usually have high levels of human growth hormones which is found in the feed of animals in order to speed up growth. This ends up in our lunch and on our dinner table. Eating of flesh and animal by-products can lead to Uterine Fibroids. Tumors are mucus that has accumulated and crystallized in the womb due to a diet of dairy, flesh and white flour.

Other related dis-eases: Menstrual Cramps, Heavy Bleeding, Clotting During Menses, PMS, Mood Swings, Vaginal Itching, Vaginal Burning, Vaginitis, Difficult Child Birth, Toxemia during pregnancy, Vaginal Cysts.

African American Statistics: Fibroids are more common among women of African-American descent. Some statistics indicate that up to 80% of African-American women will develop uterine fibroids

Spanish American Statistics: Hispanic women residing in the United States have twice the incidence rate of and 1.4 times the mortality rate from cervical cancer compared with non-Hispanic Whites

American Statistics: Approximately 20-40% of women 35 years and older have fibroid tumors

Global Statistics: For every 10,000 hysterectomies performed, 11 women die. (Approximately 660 women die each year in the United States from complications of hysterectomy.)

Womb Wellness Breath Work: With mouth closed, breathe deeply into your abdomen expanding the diaphragm, continue breathing and expanding up to the chest. Exhale fully as the abdomen contracts and the lungs release your breath completely. Practice fire breaths for a few times slowly. Then do 50 rapid fire breaths. If you begin to hyperventilate, breathe into a paper bag (not plastic) for few minutes to restore your natural breathing pattern.

Womb Affirmation: I release all toxic foods, negative thoughts, abusive/toxic relationships, self abuse and attitudes that cause a painful womb life. I embrace live

(EMPOWERMENT)

– 12 –

WOMB WELLNESS FIBROID FREE EMPOWERMENT CIRCLE WHEEL FOR FIBROID TUMOR PREVENTION

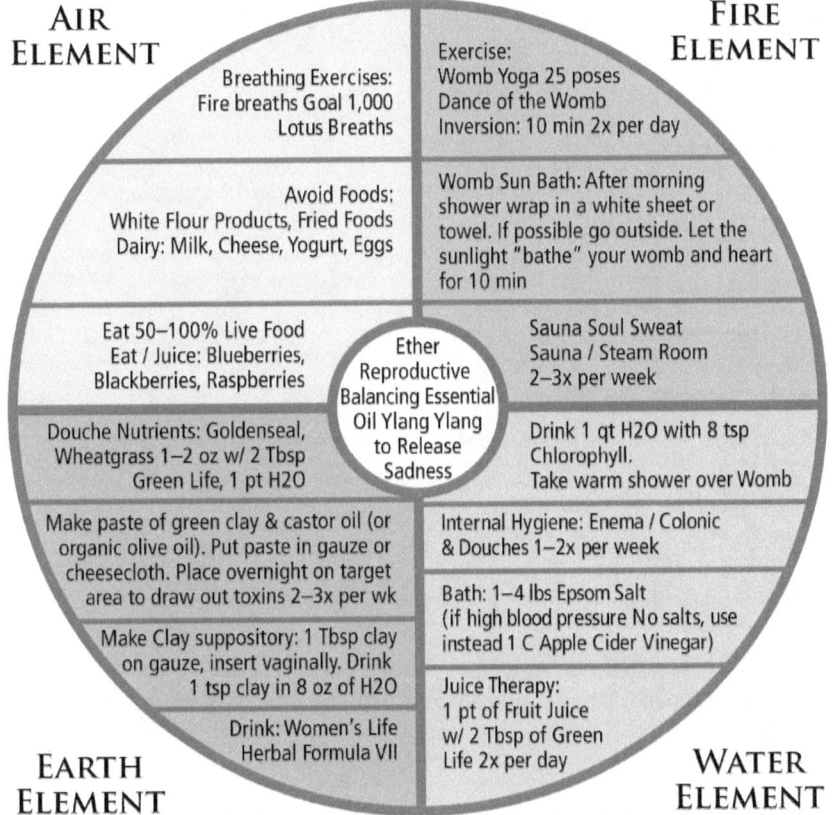

vibrant foods, positive thoughts and healthy, loving relationships and an elevated attitude which creates a healthy disease-free womb life; that I may birth healthy visions and attract healthy relationships.

Disclaimer: The information in this chart offers wellness recommendations and suggestions, and is not intended to diagnose or prescribe. Please consult with your medical physician regarding your health.

Food As Medicine

(Plants, Herbs and Elements)

NUTRITION:

Vegetarian Protein Choices:

Beans, Peas, Lentils, Raw Soaked Nuts, Raw Seeds, Sprouts, Spirulina

Sweeteners:

Soaked Dates, Raisins or Currants

Lose Weight:

At lunch and dinner consume foods and juices in order of appearance, starting with salad.

Gain weight:

Reverse the order. Start with protein.

Assist your dietary shift:

Avoid sugar, flesh, fried foods, GMO foods, micro-waved and fast foods.

For 100% live food eaters:

Convert steamed foods into a "live" dish using a food processor.

Eat organic foods whenever possible.

Enhance vegetable and protein dishes:

Use sage, oregano, parsley, bay leaf, dill, peppermint leaves, chives, rosemary leaves

A FEW MORE THINGS...about using plants, herbs and elements...

REJUVENATION BATHS:

(DO NOT USE BATH SALTS if you have HIGH BLOOD PRESSURE! Instead use Organic Apple Cider Vinegar.)

Epsom Salts:
1-4 lbs. seven nights straight; then four times a week. Soak time 15-30 minutes, then shower.

Or

Dead Sea Salts:
1lb. 1-4 lbs. seven nights straight; then, four times a week. Soak time 15-30 minutes, then shower.

INTERNAL CLEANSING:

Enemas:
3 times per week. Herbal Laxatives 3 tablets are taken every other day.

Colonics:
1-3 during the 21 Day fasting period.

Herbal Laxatives:
Take 3 tablets a day every other day.

PHYSICAL ACTIVITY:

Follow instructions from activity for 15-30 minutes daily.

100 Fire breaths 2-3x daily.

Meditation 5-15 minutes daily.

NUTRIENT SUPPLLEMENTS:

Vitamin C– 1000mg, 1T Lecithin, 2T Spirulina

Vitamin B Complex 50 mg, 1 oz. wheatgrass (optional)

Breath of Life (optional) - 3 drops 2x a day with warm water, particularly during hay-fever season.

The Benefits Of Green Life Formula I

A Closer Look at Green Life Formula I
Ingredients: Spirulina, Wheatgrass, Psyllium Husk, Flaxseed

Nutritional Contents: Spirulina, Wheatgrass, Psyllium Husk, Flaxseed, Vitamins A, B1, B2 – Folic Acid, B3-Chlorine, B5-inositol, B6 ,B1, B17 (The entire B Complex). Vitamins C (ascorbic acid) E, F, I, Potassium, Copper, Iron, Calcium, Chromium, Magnesium, Manganese, Sodium, Zinc, Phosphorus, Selenium, Cobalt, Sulfur and Trace Minerals, Vegetarian Iron & protein

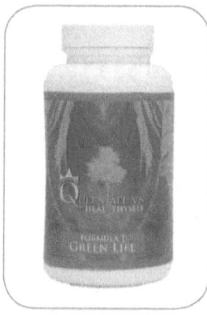

To rejuvenate your circle of wellness, each participant should ingest 2 teaspoons of Green Life Formula I, two to three times a day with fresh vegan fruit juice for your liquid meals. This should be taken 30 minutes before your solid meal.

Benefits: This formula is an excellent source of vitamins and minerals that are needed every day. This formula, when mixed with water, juice or added into a smoothie provides the body with a natural source of energy. It aids in the rejuvenation of cells, is good for assisting with high blood pressure, depression, fatigue, dizziness, fainting, headaches, and strengthening blood and bones. It also aids in weight loss.

A Closer Look at Spirulina: Spirulina is a blue-green sea algae that grows in salty lakes in Africa and Mexico. Spirulina contains B vitamins, beta carotene, Calcium, Iron, Magnesium Potassium, Manganese, and Zinc. Dried Spirulina is high in protein. Spirulina activates the immune system, counters allergic reactions, helps to protect the liver from toxic chemicals, reduces blood pressure and helps to control ulcers.

A Closer Look at Wheatgrass: Wheatgrass can be grown almost anywhere, including in your home. Liquid wheatgrass has many benefits. Liquefied, it is broken down into seventy percent Chlorophyll, which is light energy. Wheatgrass increases stamina, reduces cravings, improves fertility, aids digestion and stimulates tissue regeneration. It is good for cleaning acne, and scars. It helps purify the liver, neutralizes toxins in the body, and detoxifies colon walls and internal organs. It also reduces blood pressure and enhances capillaries, thereby improving blood circulation and cleansing the blood throughout the body. Wheatgrass is also good for the teeth, gums, neutralizing body odors and refreshing your breath. For Women, Wheatgrass helps to eliminate vaginal and uterine infections and infections in the cervix. Wheatgrass has vitamins C, A, B, E, and K as well as enzymes, glucose, Iron, Potassium, Magnesium, Calcium, Selenium, and Zinc. Wheatgrass has eight essential amino acids, making it a good source of protein.

A Closer Look at Psyllium Husk: Psyllium Husk is native ot North Africa, India, and Iran. It is derived from a seed known as flea wort. When applied topically it can treat skin irritations such as poison ivy, insect bites, stings, and rashes. When ingested, Psyllium aids in relieving constipation and diarrhea as well as bladder problems, high blood pressure, urinary tract infections, ulcers, dysentery, colitis, and rheumatism. Psyllium lowers blood cholesterol and pressure levels, helping to prevent heart disease, diabetes, and hypoglycemia. Psyllium reacts with the body, to give a feeling of fullness, which can reduce overeating and thus aid in weight loss.

A Closer Look at Flaxseed: Flaxseeds are known to have been cultivated in ancient Egypt and China. They come from flax, one of the oldest fiber crops in the world. Flaxseeds (also called linseeds) are a rich source of micronutrients, dietary fiber, manganese, vitamin B1, and the essential fatty acid alpha-linolenic acid, also known as ALA or omega-3. Omega3 support the anti-inflammatory system and lignans to help reduce the risk of breast and pancreatic cancers. Flaxseed is a source of healthy at, antioxidants, and fiber. Modern research has found evidence suggesting that flaxseed can also help lower the risk of diabetes, cancer, and heart disease.

GREEN CLAY – 21 WAYS

Rejuvenation Clay Formula V is a body food made up of calcium, magnesium, potassium, and zinc. Clay can be used internally and externally. Clay Application: Generously apply clay over area cover with gauze, allow clay to dry thoroughly. To remove clay use warm water from shower, bath or sink, wipe or sponge off with warm wet washcloth.

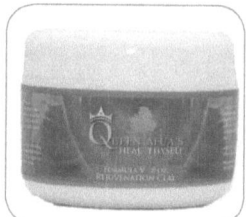

	Anatomy	Benefits	Application Time	How to use
1.	Scalp	Itchy Scalp, Hair Loss	2-3 hrs/overnight	Wash hair with natural, damp dry hair, apply and massage into hair, cover with white towel
2.	Face	Pimples, blackheads, toxic age lines	30 minutes	Wash face with warm water, dry and apply clay
3.	Eyes	Red eyes, puffy eyes, tired eyes	1-2 hours	Apply clay with eye gauze
4.	Ears	Faint hearing, ear wax build-up.	Overnight	Apply gauze behind and in front of ear
5.	Gums	Bleeding gums, gum disease	5-10 minutes	Pack a tablespoon of clay over gums, massage and rinse
6.	Teeth	Plaque/bacteria build-up	3 minutes	Brush teeth with clay as a natural toothpaste
7.	Thyroid	Enlarged thyroid	Overnight	Apply with gauze

8.	Bones & Joints	Shoulders, elbows, hands, hip bones, knees, ankles, feet	Overnight	Apply with gauze
9.	Lungs	Asthma, shortness of breath	Overnight	Apply with gauze over lungs
10.	Boils	Draws out mucus	Overnight	Apply with gauze over boils
11.	Breast	Breast tumors, cysts		Apply with gauze over breast
12.	Kidneys	Water Retention	4 hours	Apply with gauze over kidneys
13.	Womb	Pain, fibroid tumors, cysts, Vaginal Discharge, itching	Overnight or 2 hours	Apply with gauze over womb area Insert 1 teaspoon of clay with cotton swab
14.	Liver	Assists in cleansing of blood	Overnight	Apply with gauze over the liver
15.	Bladder	Soothes urinary inflammation	4 hours	Apply with gauze over the bladder
16.	Feet	Pulls toxins trapped in the body out through sweat glands of feet	Overnight	Wrap feet or toes with clay
17.	Internal Use	Pain throughout the body	Blend and drink	Blend 1 tablespoon with 8 oz. of water/juice
18.	Hand	Rejuvenates, softens	Overnight	Apply with gauze over

19.	Male Genitals	Draws out bacteria	Overnight	Apply with gauze over
20.	Skin	Promotes radiance; assists in cleansing pimples, blackheads	30 minutes	Massage clay into skin with loofa brush or sponge
21.	Sinus	Clears sinus blockage	30 minutes	Apply over sinus

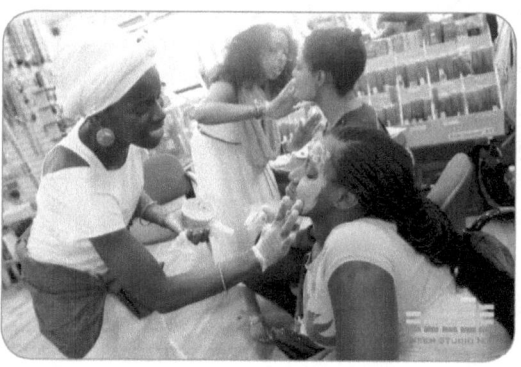

These products are not intended to be substitutes for medical prescriptions. They and the information provided are designed to help you to make informed decisions about a holistic lifestyle. If you have a medical situation, we urge you continue to follow advice prescribed by your doctor.

(EMPOWERMENT)

BREATHE, AGAIN

I never intended to become a healer or an entrepreneur, but sometimes the struggles we go through can lead us to our "calling." In other words, by solving a personal problem you have the opportunity to discover a tool to help yourself, as well as other people around the world.

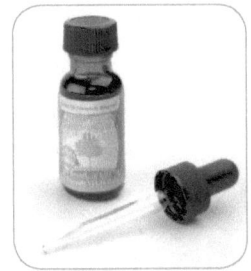

As a young woman, I suffered from asthma. I took some of the traditional remedies but to no avail. After researching various herbs, I discovered that using eucalyptus was extremely beneficial for opening up my breathing passages. Over time I learned to include dietary changes and physical exercise in my detox and purification efforts to be rid of asthma and breathe freely again.

A few months later, one of my family members called to ask me how I solved my asthma problem. That was when I realized that the herbs I had been using were the ones I would need to create the formula I would call, "Queen Afua's Breath of Spring." Since then, the name of the formula has been changed to Breath of Life Formula VI. This formula has been introduced around the globe and has brought relief from breathing challenges to many people. Supporters of Breath of Life Formula VI claim they no longer have breathing challenges, including overcoming asthma, because they use, the breath of spring that became, Breath of Life Formula VI.

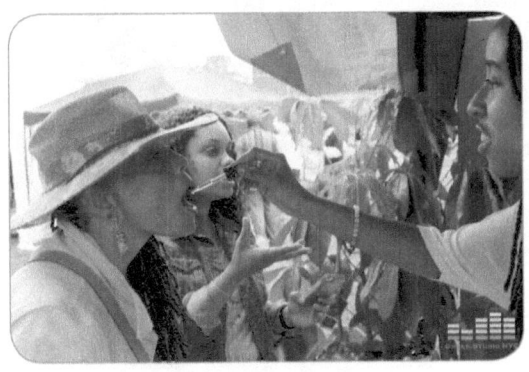

(CIRCLES OF WELLNESS)

YOUR ANATOMY, YOUR KIT

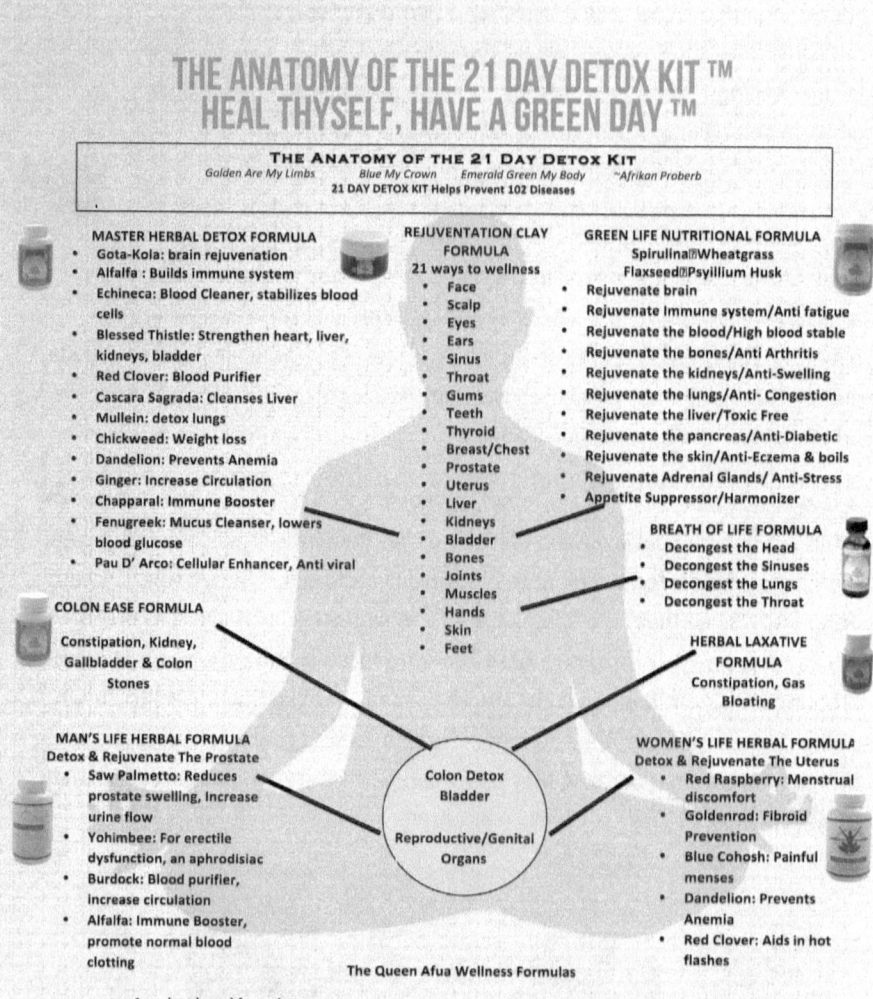

(Empowerment)

12 Points / 21 Days
Holistic Lifestyle Circles

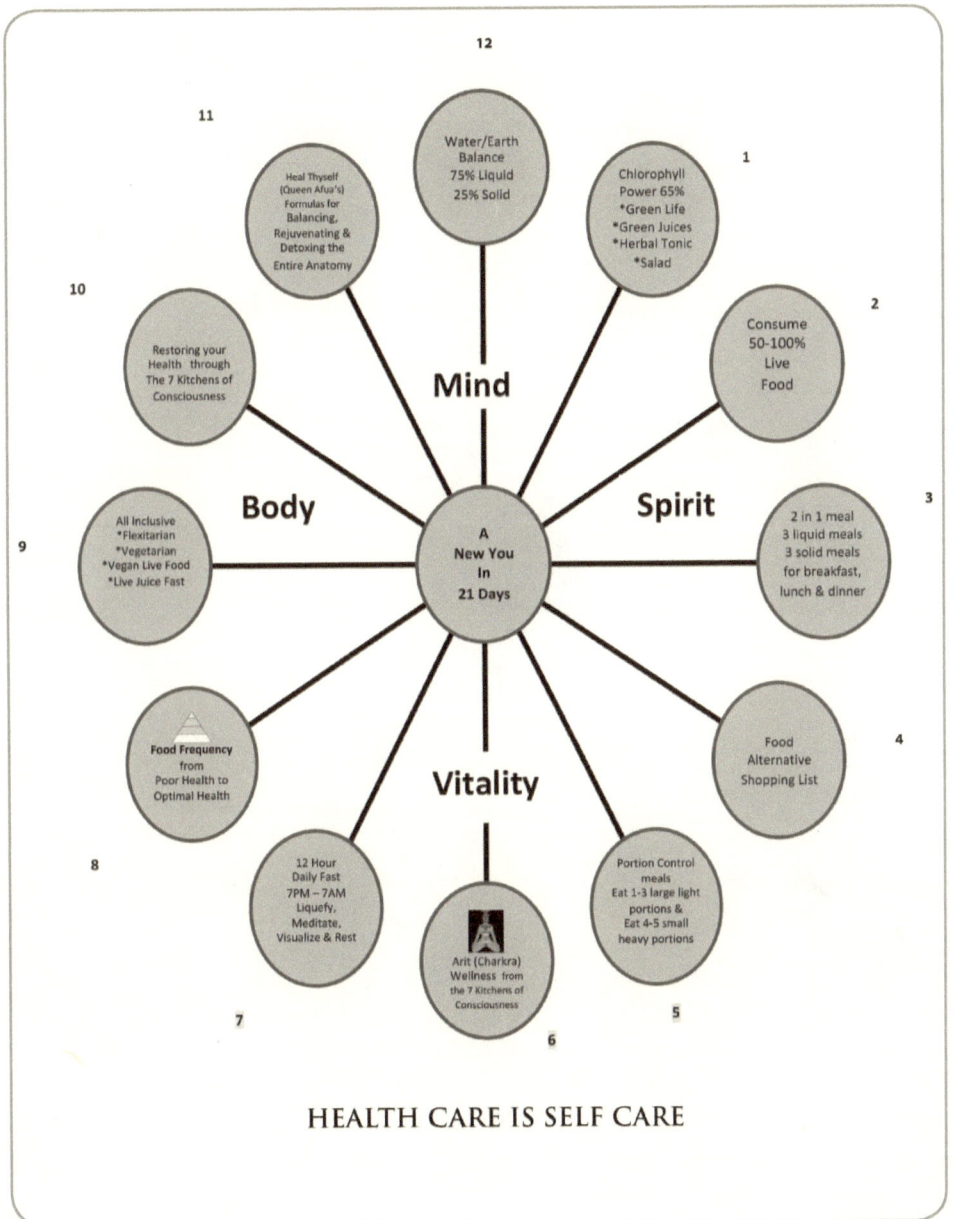

HEALTH CARE IS SELF CARE

(PARADIGM SHIFT 5)

REJUVENATION

Harvesting Wellness At Home

"Health is not only found
in hospitals and clinics.

Health care is found in homes..."

Dr. Regina M. Benjamin
United States Surgeon General (2009-2013)

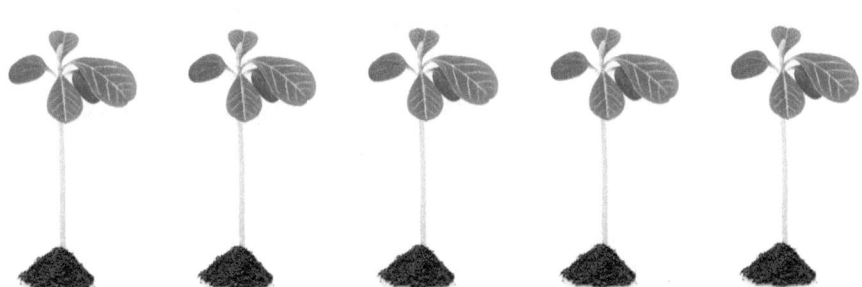

Baba Ishangi's Round House Home

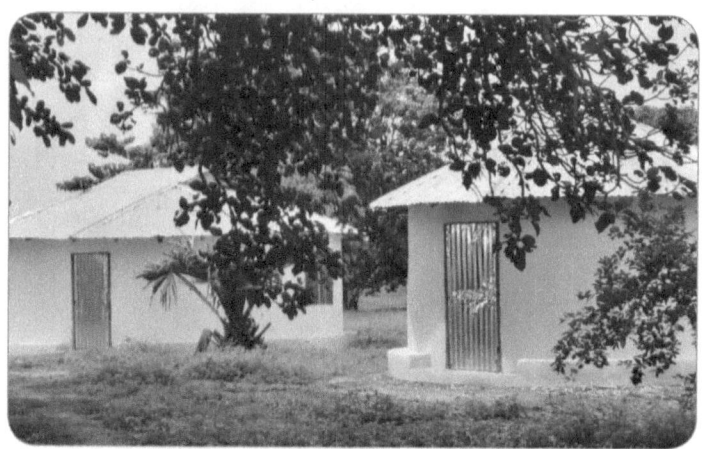

Ishangi Kunda at Banjul, Gambia, West Africa
(An Original Round House Wellness Home
Established by Baba Kwame Ishangi 1934-2003)

During Baba Ishangi's Ancestral Homecoming, Queen Afua had the honor to dwell inside of the Roundhouse he had built. Baba's final resting place is in the Round House.

"Baba Kwame Ishangi, who spiritually mentored me for over 15 years, spoke of the Round House for years. When Baba Ishangi passed, I was able to travel to the Gambia to join in the home-going service and ceremonies for sending him off to the ancestral spiritual realm. I felt honored to be on his land to be able to dwell inside The Round House he had built. The Round House represents his Cultural Healing vision and The Power of the Home to Heal. Living in Baba's Round House was a healing experience on many levels. To live in a Round House is to form a spatial Circle of Wellness that humanizes, unifies, and connects one to the Optimal Self."

*(Ishangi means keeper of the culture.)

(REJUVENATION)

SET UP YOUR WELLNESS HOME

*M*AKE A PARADIGM SHIFT. Establish a Wellness Home and you will be anchored in Wellness for the rest of your own and your family's life. Imagine each room of your home dedicated to wellness. Your home becomes your retreat for recovery; your sanctuary for serenity. Create your clinic of restoration for hope and possibility. Create your own light at the end of the tunnel; your own new beginning. Establish your Wellness Home and you will have no more sick days. In fact, you will have wellness days filled with vitality.

To have a Wellness Home each room is dedicated to specific lifestyle wellness activities which does not destroy nor diminish wellness, but rather will bring your family together in a wellness lifestyle. A Wellness Home aids the family in the prevention of disease. A Wellness Home strengthens, empowers and unifies the Family Circle. It helps keep the family engaged in healthy conversation and active connectivity filled with touchy, feely, love exchange. Together, well families can result in greater communities with calmer more positive interactions.

A Wellness Home gives a home greater purpose and reason for being. The first step to creating a Wellness Home is to de-clutter, detox, purify, wash, and clean up each room in your home. The process of Home Detoxing may take from as few as 7 days, to as many as 21 days. A Detoxed Home creates the environment for an ordered, clear mind and a harmonious spirit.

In A Wellness Home, every one, of all ages, can learn the Emerald Green 21 Day Detox Natural Healing Lifestyle Lessons. They can also learn to apply the Art of Holistic First Aid.

The second step to creating a Wellness Home is to rename the rooms in your home. The Kitchen is now renamed The Nutrition Kitchen Pharmacy where you will eat and drink food as medicine. The Bathroom is renamed the Hydrotherapy Bathroom where you will perform physical and spiritual surgery by water i.e. baths, showers, enemas, and nose rinsing using, herbs, stones, flower essences, candles and inner reflection. The Living Room is renamed the Family Live-In

CIRCLES OF WELLNESS

Room where you will perform yoga and meditation for inner peace and serenity. The Bedroom is renamed the Regeneration Bathroom where you perform regulated inversion exercises to restore your entire body from head to toe. There are Wellness Charts and Wellness Tools that will help you to create a Wellness Home.

You can use your home for personal family healing with the knowledge applied within this text. Your home can be used for conducting training lessons from the Emerald Green Level 1 Course. Also, you can expand your home into a professional wellness home with the training from the Emerald Green Level 2 Course. You can become an Emerald Green Holistic Practitioner serving your family and you community.

For over 45 years I have conducted wellness in centers and in my various homes. I have been able to serve my family and my community in Wellness. With the proper support and training and your willingness to be open and courageous, you, too can create and have an extraordinary Wellness Home.

Convert Rooms To A Wellness Home

Rooms Before Conversions	Rooms After Conversions	Wellness Conversion Charts
Kitchen	Nutrition Kitchen Pharmacy	Nutrition Kitchen chart
Kitchen	Nutrition Kitchen Pharmacy	7 Pyramids of Wellness
Kitchen	Nutrition Kitchen Pharmacy for Children	Holistic Vibrant Children Chart
Bathroom	Hydrotherapy Bathroom	Hydrotherapy Bath Spa Chart
Living Room	Live-In Room for Meditation	City of Wellness 7 Arit Meditation Chart Man Heal Thyself Scroll Sacred Woman Scroll Womb Wisdom Chart
Living Room	Live-In Room for Personal / Family Yoga (and Exercise)	Sun Ra Yoga Chart
Living Room	Live-In Room for Study	Wellness Books, Journals and reading and writing materials
Bed Room	Regeneration Bedroom	For Energy Inversion & Rest See Hydrotherapy Bath Spa Chart

Nutrition Kitchen Pharmacy Where Food Is Medicine

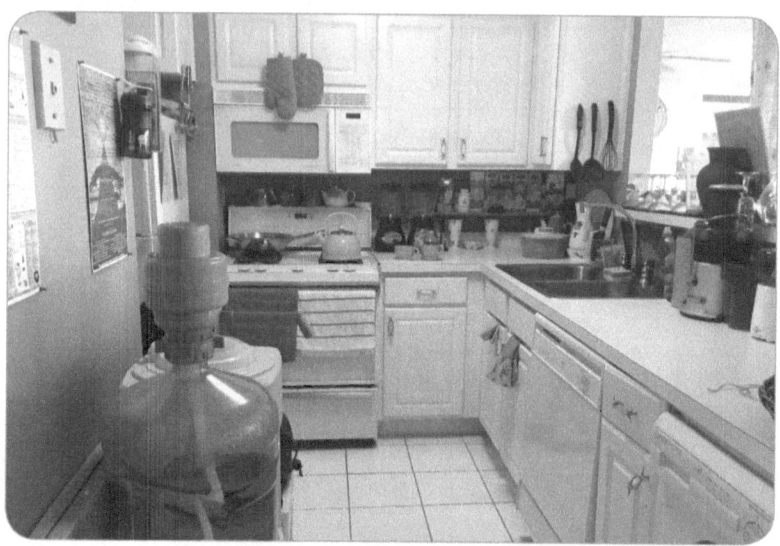

Nutrition Kitchen Pharmacy Where Food Is Medicine is the room where you use herbs, vegan proteins and whole greens to prepare salads, fruit juice smoothies and vegan soups, sauces and desserts. These delicious foods will detoxify and rejuvenate the entire anatomy in order to prevent disease and gain optimal well-being. Throughout this text you have been advised that what you eat and how you prepare it has a large impact on the state of your wellness. Constant consumption of toxic foods will create more conditions of dis-ease. On the other hand, by shifting your paradigm to include living an Emerald Green Lifestyle will help transform you toward a state of wellness in body, mind and spirit. Use your charts and texts to guide you to choose foods that can best support and nourish you and your family. Begin by setting up your kitchen to support the food preparation portion of your journey toward wellness.

My Kitchen Is Free From Negativity

My kitchen is free from negativity.
It's Serious business, my kitchen Healing Laboratory.
I sit at the crossroad, cast-iron pot in right hand and Bush Tea in my left,
I check all bags and boxes for contents of death.
I awaken the sleeping, rejuvenate the living, energize and purify
with soups and tonics, live foods, and juices.
No death in here, no chickens, no pigs, no cows or lamb.
No fish, no goats, no milk, no ham.
It's plain to see that what we eat can make us free.
Beware, for some of what binds and holds us
still comes in many forms and fashions.
It's resting right there on your plate.

Dead foods control our Mood swings.
Family fights, husbands, wives, children too.
We eat our war so, violence rings.
Yes, we do.
We hold the weapons of death right in our hands
—with forks and spoons, through pots and pans.
Beware of Mr. Flesh Burger, Dripping pizza, greasy french fries too, diet soda,
It's all sugar blues, stuff we simply cannot use.
Beware the habit, beware the ruse, the perfect program to make you lose.

Demons wrapped so beautifully, stopping us from who we really be.
Demons, demons, Get out of my healing laboratory, get out of my pot.
Causing putrefaction and rot.
It's sunrise sausages, coffee and cream,
It's bedtime cookies and cow's ice cream.
I'll wash you out and set you free
For purification is the key.
Check your kitchen cabinets, those bags and boxes too.
If' it's not live, it's not coming through.

(CIRCLES OF WELLNESS)

Fruits, vegetables, nuts, whole grains, you're all welcome to remain.
Regain your mind, your nerves, your flesh,
your bones, your breast, your knees, your chest.
Regain your husband and your children, release the strife,
As you chase the demons from your Life.
Restore your Kitchen Healing Laboratory with power, pride, and dignity.
You hold the power within your hand To raise the dead and free the land
Flesh free, drug and alcohol free, processed food and sugar free
Is how the kitchen becomes a Healing Laboratory.

Poem by Queen Afua
from *Sacred Woman*

MODEL AND TOOLS

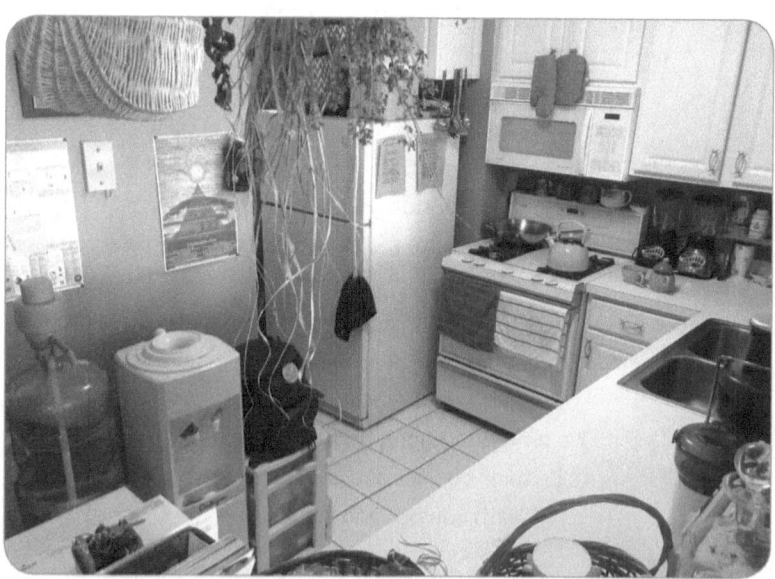

Display Wellness Charts:
Nutrition Kitchen Chart, 7 Pyramids of Power Chart, Children Holistic Chart

On the counter:
From 21 DAY DETOX KIT
- Green Life Formula I (add to juices)
- Master Herbal Formula II (for detox tea)
- Woman's Life Formula VII (for detox tea)
- Manpower Formula VIII (for detox tea)
- Colon Ease Formula III
- Herbal Laxative IV
- Breath of Life Formula VI (can also be kept in hydrotherapy room)

Herbs and Spices
- Dill
- Marjoram
- Cayenne
- Sage
- Ginger
- Sea salt

Food Preparation Tools:
- Blender
- Juicer
- Food Processor
- Stainless Steel Pots
- Tea Strainer
- Dehydrator
- Water Purifier

On the Stove:
Master Herbal Tonic (Steeping overnight)

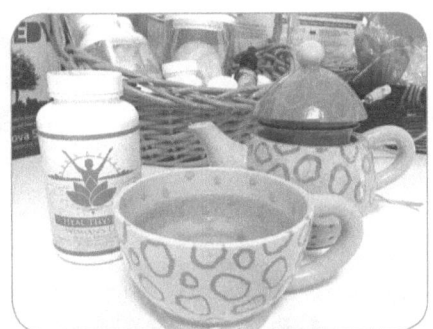

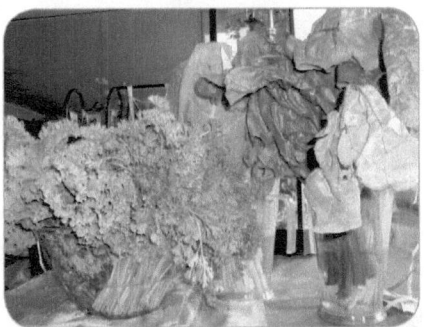

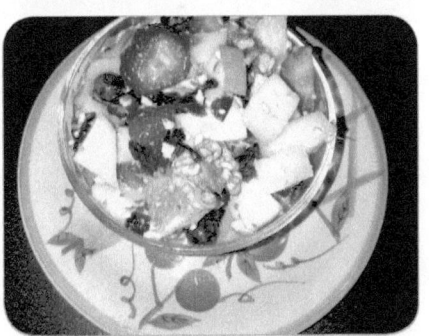

In the "Green" Refrigerator
Fresh, organic produce

On the table:
Fresh organic fruit for snacks

(CIRCLES OF WELLNESS)

AN INVITATION

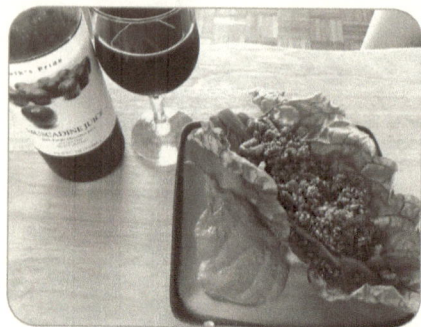
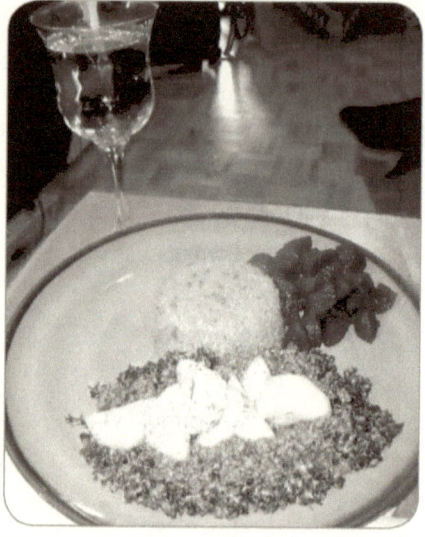
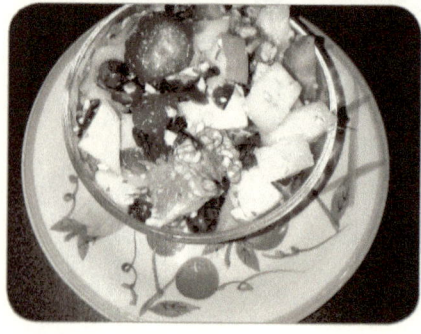

Lunch: BBQ Savory Wrap, Homemade Green Goddess Dressing, Organic Grape Juice;
Dinner: Kale, Cucumber, Beets, Seed Loaf;
Dessert: Mango Pudding (From Sacred Woman Auset Aswad's Nutrition Kitchen)

You are invited to the
Nutrition Kitchen Pharmacy
hosted by
The Global Nation of Wellness & The People's Chef Ali Amechi.
I have set the table.
I have laid out a delicious life–affirming
spread to feed your body in order to once again create a living temple.
Partake until you are filled.
Fortify your life with each scrumptious bite.
The who's who will be attending
Breakfast, Lunch, Dinner.
Don't miss out on this healthy company.
You are more than welcome to regain your vitality from Nature's Pharmacy.

LET'S DINE!

(REJUVENATION)

WHOLE FOOD AFFIRMATION

I peacefully prepare whole foods from the Nutrition Kitchen Pharmacy that feed and reflect love and inner harmony; restoring every cell, muscle bone and nerve. Through holistic consumption I ingest health and longevity. I embrace and bless whole foods from nature's garden to fortify and purify me. May I, a Citizen of Wellness, release the chains from the toxic fast food Corporate Kitchens that I may cleanse, elevate and empower myself through the 7 Kitchens of Consciousness. May whole foods from nature's pharmacy transform me into a pure body temple of wellness from dis-ease. May I overcome all toxic food addictions and become a beacon of wellness, thereby radiating health and wholeness to all of my friends and family. With a peaceful mind, a calm spirit and open heart I prepare whole foods daily to uplift and rejuvenate my inner frequency.

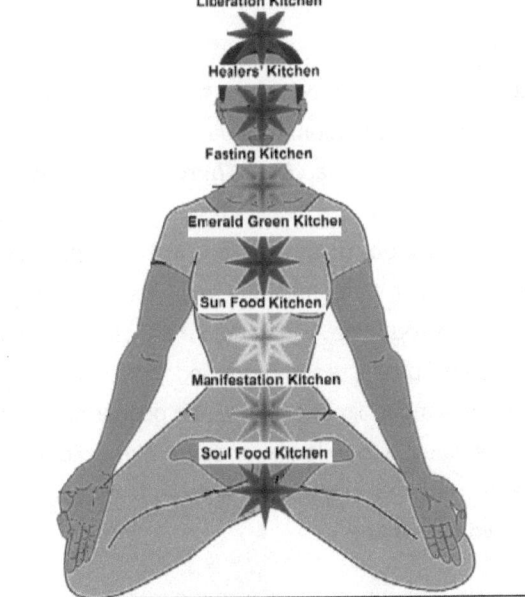

For over 250 delicious and vibrant vegan recipes for healthy living review the text, **City of Wellness** and explore within it the 7 Kitchens of Consciousness.

(CIRCLES OF WELLNESS)

The following is from a mother who converted her kitchen to a Nutrition Kitchen Pharmacy. She was able to heal her child from a chronic asthma condition.

A Mother's Testimony

Greetings, I want to let you know Queen Afua is the TRUTH!! I became acquainted with Queen's teachings in 1994. My son, 3 years old at the time, had been suffering from asthma since he was 6 months old. We were in the ER every weekend .The medical bills were huge and the prescriptions were expensive. Doctors told me my son had severe asthma, was allergic to everything and would have to spend most of his life inside. One night when he was having a severe attack the doctors gave him several treatments and a shot, but nothing was working. They admitted him and put him in an isolation tent. When they finally discharged him the doctors prescribed an adult inhaler (Albuterol) as the only way they could treat him. They admitted that it was filled with steroids and told me how the side effects would affect my son's quality of life. I was devastated...

I brought my baby home and I started talking to everyone about asthma. They all said – he needs to take medication. One day I expressed my frustration to a friend who suggested that I read **Heal Thyself** by Queen Afua. In the introduction Queen shared her own healing from asthma and allergies. Maybe I had found an answer. I scheduled a phone consultation with Queen Afua. When we talked I explained my son's situation. She said, "Beloved, your son will be okay. This is what I need you to do..." She told me that I needed to immediately eliminate all dairy, animal products and processed food. Queen told me to let my son fast on grapefruit, lemons, limes and cayenne pepper for two days. She said to give him plenty of water, and to love him, touch him, hold him, sing to him and to affirm that he is healed. I remember saying, "No food? He's just a baby," Queen said he would be just fine.

So, I did everything she told me to do. I juiced the fruit. I gave him water and the juice mixture for two days. I held him. I affirmed his healing to myself and to him. I started saying, "Thank you for healing my son." My baby cried and cried. All of a sudden he had to use the bathroom. Oh, my God, the toilet was filled

(Rejuvenation)

with mucus! My son was coughing and sneezing up large amounts of mucus. Mucus was coming from his eyes, nose and ears – just everywhere! I continued to give him the drink Queen had recommended. After two days there was no more mucus. My son slept all day the 3rd day. On the 4th day he was playful. His eyes were very clear and bright. There was no wheezing, no coughing. He was full of energy! It was just wonderful! I thought, let me test this. We walked to the corner store. There were no episodes. An entire week went by and he didn't have an asthma attack. Overjoyed, I called Queen to thank her and let her know what had happened. She told me to get some Red Clover tincture and put a couple of drops in his water to purify his blood. I did that…

At my son's follow-up doctor's appointment they took an x-ray and listened to his chest. There was no wheezing; his lungs were clear. Of course the doctors attributed this to their medicine. I told them I had never filled the prescription. I told them step by step what I had done. The doctor told me whatever I was doing is working, so continue. I told my family the great news. They threatened to call Children's Services on me for neglect if I didn't give my son the medicine and stop this food "craziness". I told them they could call whomever they wanted. My son was healed. He could go outside and play and not spend weekends in the ER. He could participate in physical activity without feeling like he's going to die.

That was 22 years ago. My son is now an adult and never had another asthma attack. No allergies. No inhaler. Nothing. He is just fine and it's all because I changed our diet. We both became vegan. My son still juices daily, lemons, grapefruits, limes and cayenne pepper. Food is his medicine. Thank you, Queen Afua, you taught me how to change the way I live and you saved my son's life. I love you eternally for that.

(CIRCLES OF WELLNESS)

HYDROTHERAPY BATHROOM

Where Water Surgery
Is For Balancing and Harmonizing

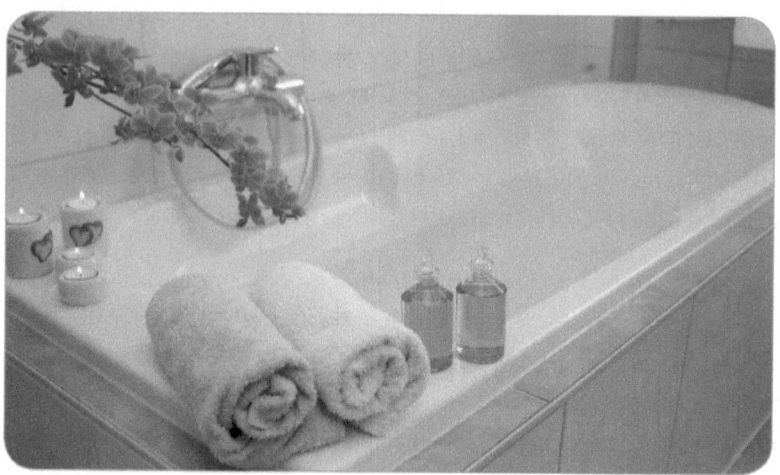

The Hydrotherapy Bathroom is the room where through "water surgery" one detoxifies and rejuvenates the entire anatomy. By taking salt and herbal baths, showers, enemas, and performing nose-rinsing one can prevent disease and gain radiant, serene, well-being. Make your bathroom your nature sanctuary; your water surgery home spa (bathroom) for body, mind and soul harmony. For maximum wellness, take a Therapeutic Hydrotherapy Bath everyday for 28 days, then 2 – 3x per week as a way of life.

Harmonize Your Mind • Purify Your Body
Renew Your Spirit • Balance Your Relationships

Display Wellness Chart:

Hydrotherapy Bath Spa Chart

Following are highlights from the Hydrotherapy Bath Spa Chart.

Hydrotherapy Tools:
- Loofah Brush/ Sea Weed Sponge Dry Brush
- Squatting Stool
- Enema Bag
- Live Plant for Window
- Waterpik for Dental Care
- Hand Held Shower/Whirlpool Bath
- Potpourri
- Foot Stone
- Rejuvenation Clay & Breath of Life Colon Ease & Herbal Laxatives
- Oatmeal Scrub
- Organic Liquid Soap
- Massage Oil

Therapeutic Hydrotherapy Baths:
Choose one of the following baths to support your wellness:

Sitz Bath, Salt Bath, Apple Cider Vinegar Bath, Master Herbal Bath, Circulation Bath, De-Stress Herbal Bath

De-Stress Herbal Bath:
Boil 3 cups of water, turn off flame then add 3 teaspoons of chamomile & hops, cover and soak overnight or for 4 hours, strain and add to bath. If you DO NOT have high blood pressure, add 2 lbs. of Epsom salt or Dead Sea Salt to the warm water bath. Soak for 20 – 30 minutes then follow up with alternate temperature shower. DO NOT USE SALT if you have HIGH BLOOD PRESSURE, instead, take Apple Cider Vinegar Bath.

Hydro-tonics:
Drink 1 of the following tonics while bathing. The Flusher, The Mucous Cleanser, The Rejuvenator, The Detoxifier

The Mucous Cleanser: Add juice of 1 Lemon/Lime to 8 – 16 oz. of H2O

Alternate Temperature Shower or Bath:

Focused Therapeutic Alternative Temperature Bath – Increase your circulation and wake up your skin. Wash the skin to release poisons through the pores. Run water over entire body warm to hot, then cool to cold 1– 3 times while massaging your body from head to toe with loofah brush, seaweed sponge or with your hands in a clockwise circular motion to align your energy with universal power.

Full Body Alternate Temperature Shower - For Focused Hydrotherapy, use a showerhead to direct water over specific area that you are treating Shower, alternating temperatures from hot to cold for 10 seconds, 2 – 3 times over focus area.

Intimate Hydrotherapy:

This work can be performed individually to enhance relationships with self, or as a couple to strengthen relationships with your significant other. Intimate Hydrotherapy can be done for: Organic Oral Hygiene, Head-to-Toe Application, Sinus Detox, Colon Detox, Douche (Vaginal Detox), Prostate Clay Pack

Hot Castor Oil H2O Pack:

Overall, most needed to soften the hard impacted toxic body member. Boil water and dip a clean flannel or white wash cloth into the water. Wring out the cloth, saturate it with cold-pressed castor oil and place over pelvic area.

Cover top of cloth with plastic wrap then apply a heating pad for one hour. Remove castor oil pack and apply thick clay pack overnight.

For Hydrotherapy Tools: Charts, Aromatherapy Mist & Bath Salts, Hydrotherapy Bathroom Workshop & Anti Pain Consultation Call (888)-344-HEAL for Queen Afua, creator & producer of The Holistic Hydrotherapy Bathroom Home Spa

Family Live-In Room

For Meditation/Study/Exercise & Yoga
For Inner Peace

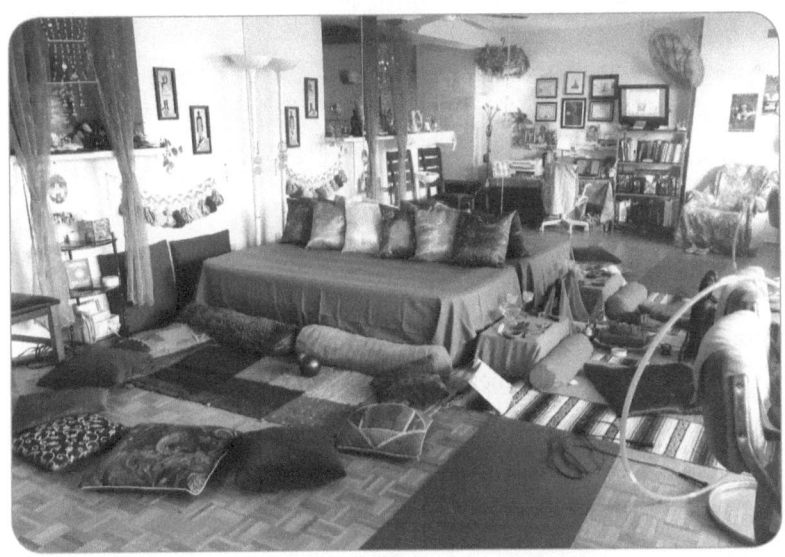

The Family Live-In Room is a multi-purpose room for Meditation, Study, Creativity, Exercise, and Yoga. You can meditate away stress and practice movements such as yoga to relieve tension and create inner strength and harmony. Use this room to reserve daily quite time and to study wellness lessons, write in your journal, and to tap into your "Inner Vision through Wellness Journey." The Live-In Room is where you can get in touch and in-tuned with yourself. Typically, living room is often used as a television room where people "numb out" their mind and heart from a stress-filled, toxic day or even life. Let the tranquility of the Live-In Room inspire you to create Inner Vision and Inner-tainment that supports wellness and joy.

>"I GO IN TO COME TO LIFE...."
>**The African Proverbs**

Live-In Room Vision Quest & Meditation Corner

Display Live-In Room Charts:
- 7 Arit Meditation Chart
- Man Heal Thyself Scroll
- Sacred Woman Scroll
- Womb Wisdom Chart
- Sun Ra Yoga Chart

Study Tools:
- Wellness Books & CDs
- Journal

Meditation Tools:
- Green Candle for Regeneration/ Rejuvenation
- White Candle for Clarity
- Music/musical Instruments

Set up an area or corner in your Live-in Room to serve as your meditation and vision quest space. Include in the area a small table to hold your wellness

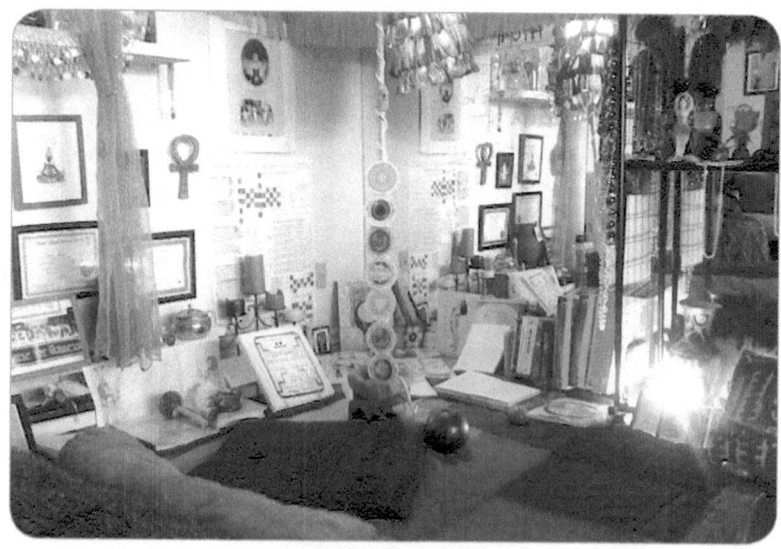

(REJUVENATION)

journal, your wellness texts and study materials, such as Heal Thyself and City of Wellness. You might also include a white candle for clarity and a green candle for regeneration and rejuvenation. In this space you can read, meditate and write in your journal.

Affirm: I am a healer. I am healing myself and all my relations, as I heal myself.

LIVE-IN ROOM EXERCISE AREA

Exercise Tools:
- Stationary bike
- Light weights
- Jump rope
- Hula hoop
- Fitness ball

Set up an area in your Live-in Room to use fitness equipment and/or to do Yoga and exercises for Optimal Wellness.

Celebrate your Wellness!

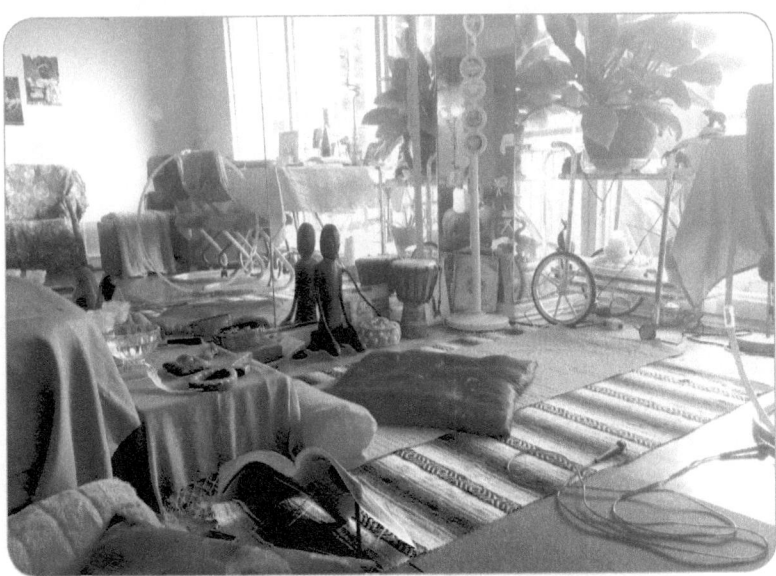

Sun Ra Yoga

"The Mystery of the Hidden Sun Is Revealed To My Face"

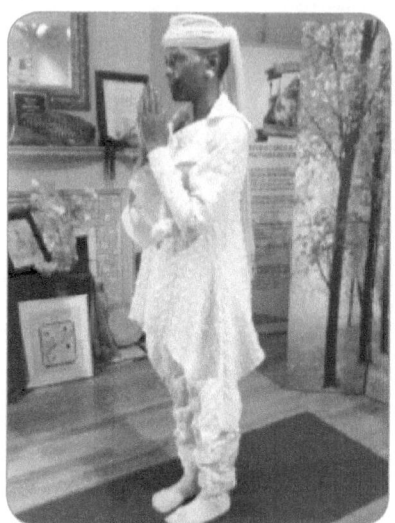

1. Sunrise Center Pose

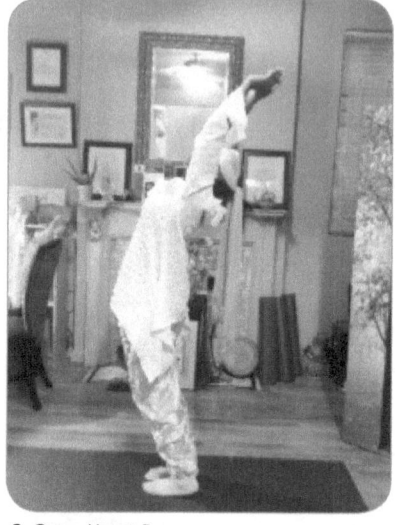

2. Open Heart Pose

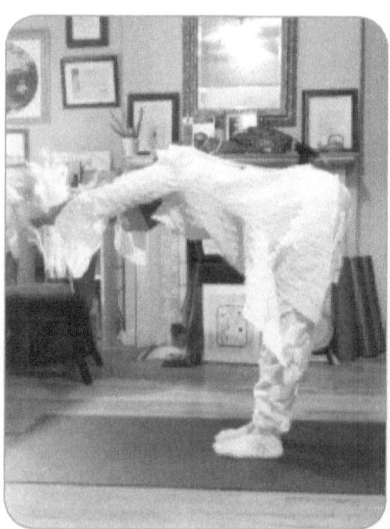

3. Flat Back Pose

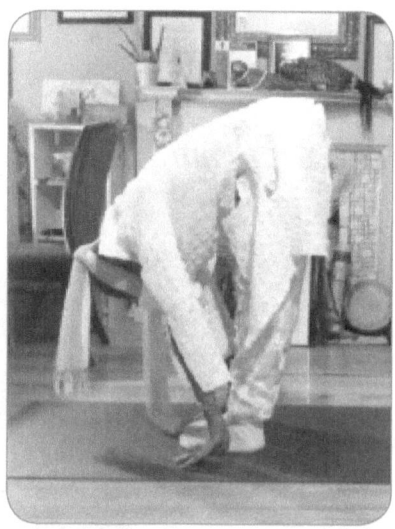

4. Sunset Pose

Rejuvenation

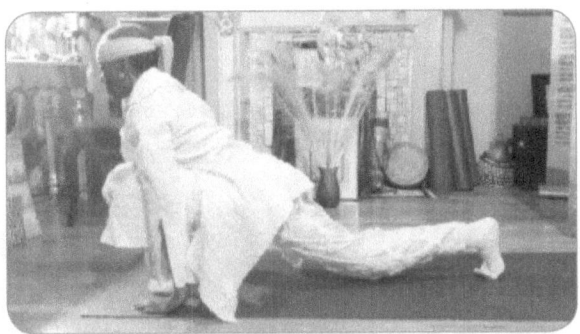

5. Forward Stretch Pose

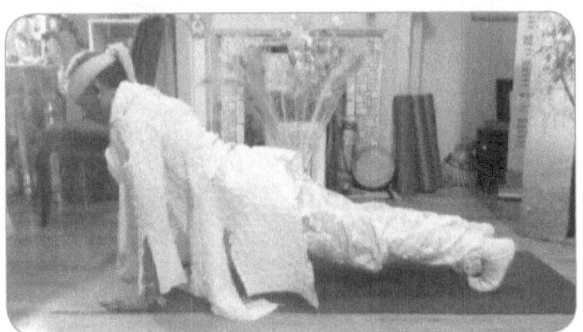

6. Advanced Back Leg Pose

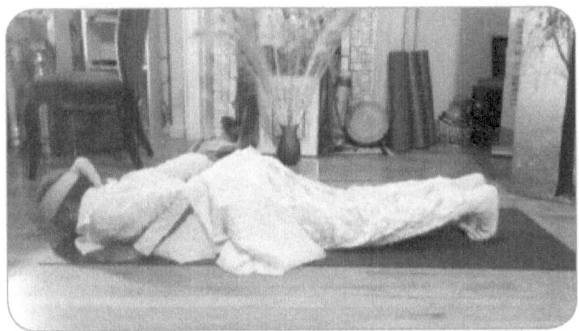

7. Surrender Pose

(CIRCLES OF WELLNESS)

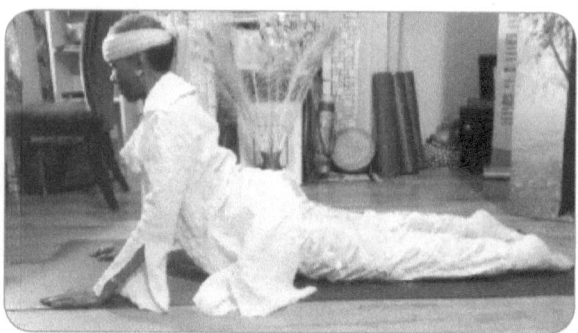

8. Cobra Pose

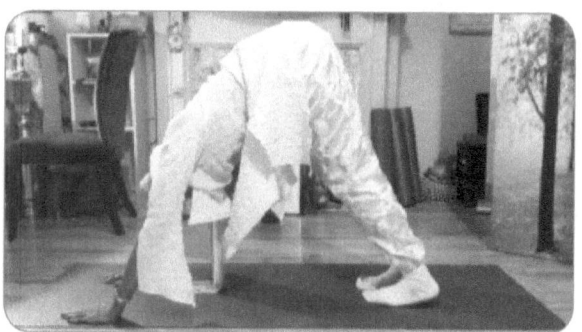

9. Pyramid Pose

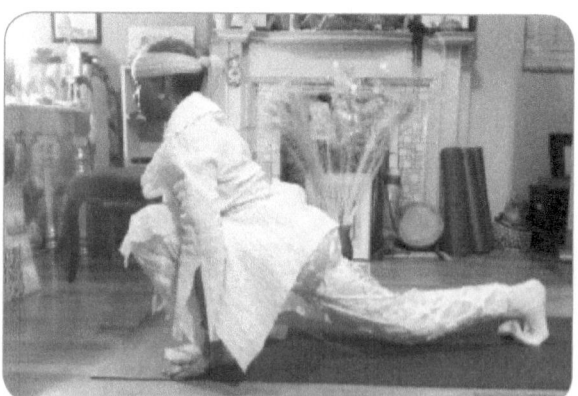

10. Forward Stretch Pose

(Rejuvenation)

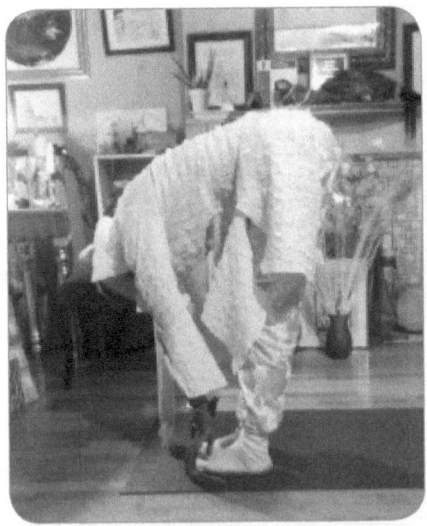

11. Sunset Pose

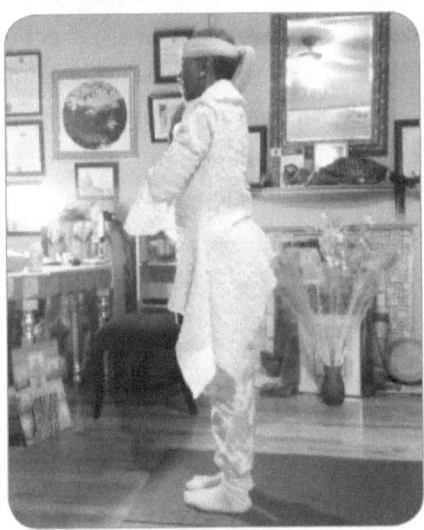

12. Sunrise Pose

The Regeneration Bedroom

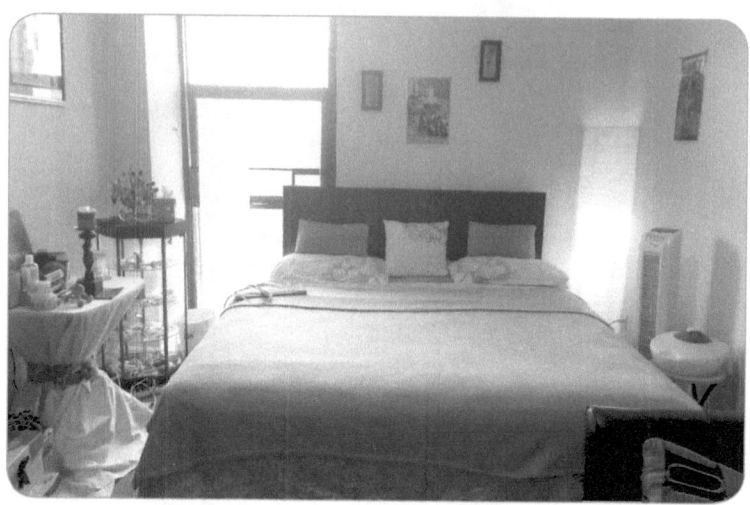

The Regeneration Bedroom is your center for alignment and rest. by performing Inversion Therapy daily, you can flush all blockages from the circulatory system as you realign your entire anatomy. Daily practice of Inversion Therapy helps you to maintain a youthful body temple. When decorating your Regeneration Bedroom choose colors, fabrics, scents, and sounds that will support your peace of body, mind and spirit. Couples regard and maintain your Regeneration Bedroom as a sanctuary for harmonious, healing, and holistic lovemaking.

> "I AM IN THE UJAD OF HIGHER CONSCIOUSNESS.
> I GO IN TO COME TO LIFE"
> ~African Proverb

Inversion Therapy:
Lie flat in bed or on floor then place legs in 45° angle or perform a 3 pillow lift under the legs. Breathe deep inhalations and exhalations throughout the treatment. While breathing, self message chest and abdomen with palms in a clockwise direction 7- 21 times to further breakup & dissolve blockage in the arteries; the mainstream passageway to all your major organs.

Rejuvenation

The regular practice of Inversion Therapy for 20 minutes each at Sunrise and Sunset can help you eliminate: Clogged Arteries, Congested Lungs, Poor Memory, Poor, Circulation, Constipation, Prolapsed Womb, Lower Back Pain, Dizziness, Headaches, Swelling of Ankles, Stress, Numbness, Difficulty Breathing, Gas, Sinus Congestion, and Fatigue.

Benefits of Inversion Therapy include:
- Energy • Clarity • Vitality • Serenity • Wellness
- Rejuvenation • Balance • Longevity

Benefits of Inversion Therapy
- Relieves Fatigue
- Unclogs Thoughts
- Unclogs Arteries
- Decongests the Anatomy
- Melts Away Cellulite
- Prevents Dizziness
- Relieves Constipation
- Relieves Pain Due To Blockage
- Increases Circulation
- Increases Memory
- Increases Mental Clarity
- Relaxes the Body
- Increases Digestion
- Relieves Lower Back Pain
- Improves Vision
- Detoxifies the Lungs

Rest:
Regenerate for 6 – 8 hours; do not eat any solids after hydrotherapy bath.

For optimal Wellness Days * De-stress * Relax * Rejuvenate * in your Regeneration Bedroom.

Now That You Know

1. From Paradigm Shift 1, use the Wellness Worksheets to begin planting your Circles of Wellness for all levels from personal to global.
2. From Paradigm Shift 2, examine the magnificent possibilities of holistic and allopathic circles united to plant, cultivate and harvest wellness.
3. From Paradigm Shift 3, choose dietary practices from one or all of the Nutrition Kitchen Meal Plans. From 21 days to 12 weeks follow the nutritional path that will best holistically detoxify and rejuvenate you.
4. From Paradigm Shift 4, use the Wellness Challenges Checklist for self evaluation. Check off wellness imbalances and challenges. Every 21 Days reevaluate your state of well-being on your Wellness Challenges Checklist:
   - Place an "X" next to any dis-eases have been eliminated
   - Place an "L" next to any that have lessened.
   - Keep a ✓ (check mark) next to those dis-eases / conditions with no change.
5. From Paradigm Shift 4, apply strategies found in the 12 Empowerment Wheel Circles, which best correspond to your wellness needs.
6. Purchase your 21 Day or 12 Week Detox Kit and other wellness products to support you as you detoxify and rejuvenate. (See Catalog Pages.)
7. Setup your Wellness Home based on suggestions presented in Paradigm Shift 5.

Every 21 days you can expect one of the following Wellness Paradigm Shifts:

Module 1: Day 1-21 (21 Days): 40-50% Wellness

Module 2: Day 22-42 (21 Days): 60% Wellness

Module 3: Day 43-63 (21 Days): 70% Wellness

Module 4: Day 64-84 (21 Days): 80-100% Wellness

Health Care Is Self Care

(POSTSCRIPT)

Next Steps

Global Fast

Healers' Words

Catalogue

(CIRCLES OF WELLNESS)

24 Hour Global Fast

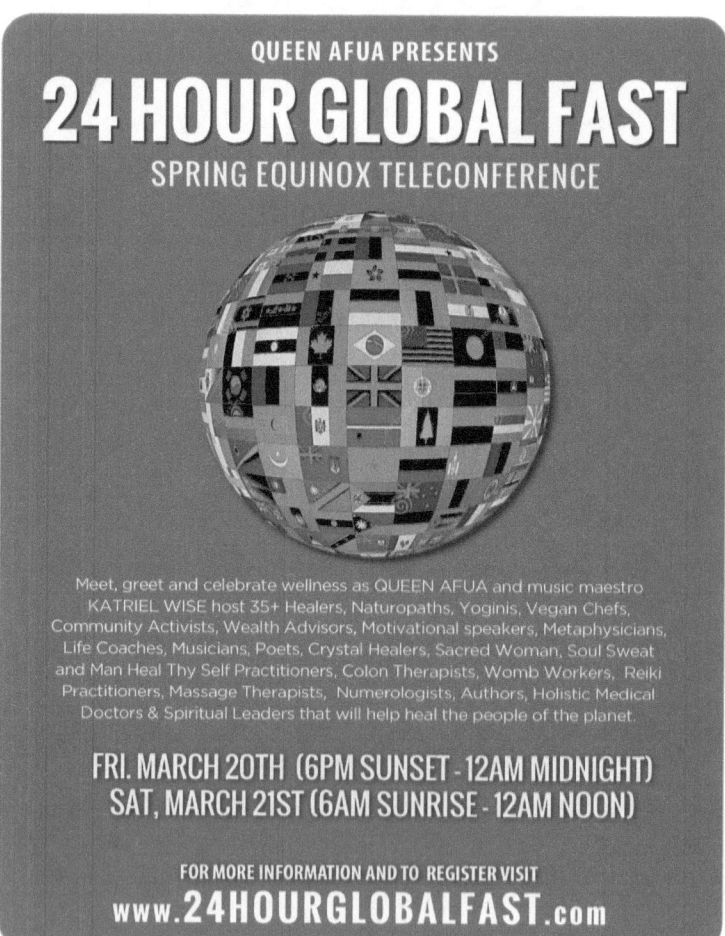

(NEXT STEPS)

CIRCLE OF HEALERS

In the spring of 2014 I was inspired to reach out to my friends in the healing community to help me launch a Nation To Nation – City to City 24 Hour Global Fast Teleconference. They came, over seventy Healers, Naturopaths, Yoginis, Vegan Chefs, Community Activists, Wealth Advisors, Motivational Speakers, Metaphysicians, Life Coaches , Musicians, Poets, Crystal Healers, Sacred Women, Soul Sweat and Man Heal Thyself Practitioners, Colon Therapists, Womb Workers, Reiki Practitioners, Massage Therapists, Numerologists, Authors, Medical Doctors and Spiritual Leaders , they came together as a Circle of Healers to send out their messages to help heal the people on our planet. Since then, the healers are convinced that if we keep gathering together, the people will come. So to the people who find themselves with these pages in their hands – COME! Join us on the Day That Healed the World.

SPRING EQUINOX
    SUMMER SOLSTICE
        FALL EQUINOX
            WINTER SOLSTICE

The first time that I experienced a mass union for a common cause I was 9 years old, in Washington, DC, standing in the mud and rain between my mother and father while listening to Martin Luther King Jr.'s "I Have A Dream" speech. I was surrounded by millions listening to greatness. Another memorable time I experienced people coming together for mass liberation was during the sixties when people from all walks of life –spiritual, economic, social, and cultural– rose up to liberate themselves. We took our walk to the streets, to our homes, from City to City. We woke up to freedom. We rode the buses and marched; and sat in -- in our homes, in our cities.

Now, throughout our nations, healers are being called on to gather to mend; to heal a broken, divided, wounded, dis-eased, hurt world. We come with the healing balm of natural medicine to free the people from harm. We, The Healers speak out for The People to resurrect, recover, overcome, detox and fast from all dead thoughts, dead actions, dead words, dead deeds and dead food. We, The People are working to raise our vibrational frequency so that we may empty the jails of our youth and empty old age homes of the elderly and move them to *Heal Thyself*. We, The People claim the right to live a life of optimal mental, physical, emotional health and longevity; peace and prosperity. We, The People are willing to work together to put down our swords against one another to save our children from a legacy of dis-ease and mass destruction. We, The People seek to achieve vibrant families and communities, vibrant neighborhoods and cities, vibrant nations in a vibrant world.

We, The People are naming and claiming ourselves Freedom Fighters for Wellness, Champions of Wholeness, and Emerald Green Riders. We, The Healers are willing to share our knowledge, our experiences, our visions, our mastery, our intelligence and our gifts of healing that we may all be well, be whole, be present; be liberated from dis-ease. We, The People are willing to align ourselves to optimal living, willing to clean up our bodies and our minds. We are willing to take responsibility for our well-being, and willing to blame no one for the choices we make of our free will. We, The People are choosing to be renewed, restored, and rejuvenated. We, The People have shifted to higher ground; we are indestructible. Not even our DNA can hold us back; nor will history deny us wholeness. This is our time to be whole; right now at this very moment.

There are thousands of us, millions of us in the world. These healers share with you. They repeat that there is a way out, a way up, a way to wellness. May you be inspired by their sharing, encouraged by their vision and charged by their walk. Let them lead you on the journey to living large, living strong, living holistically. They are a multitude of healing disciples who share their talk and walk with you that you may be whole. The following are a few of the healers.

WE ARE UNIFYING. WE ARE COMING. WE ARE HERE.

(NEXT STEPS)

HIP-HOP MEDICINE MAN

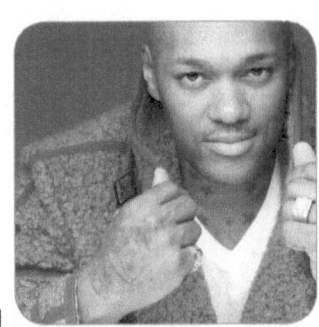

Supa Nova Slom was born in the heart of Brooklyn and spent a part of his youth on the streets of New York. He was barely a teenager when he started running with gangs and within a few years, it was clear that he would have to find a way out. He went to live with family in the South. When he returned to Brooklyn, his life really changed. He began taking his ideas for social healing back to the streets where he had grown up. Now known as The Hip-Hop Medicine Man, Supa Nova's philosophy comes from both his own experiences and the teachings of his mother, world-renowned holistic practitioner and author, Queen Afua. The vegan inspired lyrics of detoxification and purification in his music are delivered in hip-hop genre! His direct and positive message announces empowerment of self and the community, especially to the youth.

TASTES SO GOOD

Chorus (Repeat twice)
I know it's so bad, but it taste so good
It hurts so bad, but it taste so good
My uncle's big, so big he can't walk
His face is swoll, so swoll he can't talk
My auntie wheezing, she need a pump to breathe
Back an' forth, in and out of the hospital
She breathing through machines
Trying to help them both get off that junk, junk food
get with them greens
They don't really want to hear the medicine,
their addicted to them southern things
Candied yams, fat back, overcooked greens and pigs feet
You know that soul food, it won't let you go, it holds you

(CIRCLES OF WELLNESS)

Chorus (repeat twice)
My brother's diabetic, but he keeps eating candy
My sister's asthmatic, but she keeps eating dairy
Mama loves salt; high blood pressure scary
All around the hood see the fast food stores
If we don't change our diet, man we won't live long
Man we don't live long now a' days, anyway
It taste so good all these sugs in these foods
Man it keeps us coming back,
suga' crack in these foods
Chorus (repeat twice)
50,000 on my neck
20,000 on my earlobe
10,000 on my wrist
$2.00 in my stomach
I bling outside while
my insides die, nutritionally
deficient, so what I shine
drink, drink no juice
sip soda, no juice with a little codeine
'till I'm chopped up and screwed
'till my body break down man I can't stop now
They say health is wealth but am so broke now
Because it taste so good we sick up in the hood
Am addicted to the sickness man
It's all through the hood
Cause it taste so good, we sick up in the hood,
Am addicted to this sickness
Man it's all through the hood
Chorus (repeat twice)

Nova's mantra is:
"The Wellness Warrior Creed is: Purify or Die."

Visit Nova on his website
www.WellnessSalute.com

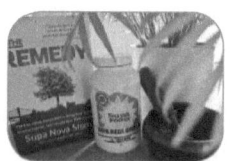

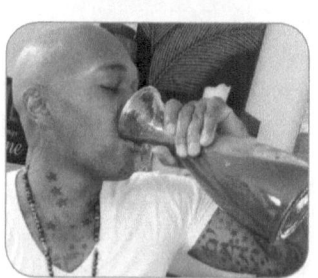

(Next Steps)

CROP CIRCLES

Collectively, as Healers of this Planet Earth, we are forming a force field of Spiritual Crop Circles. When we study the Crop Circles found and formed in various parts of this Planet, we discover that something amazing occurs within the interior of these Celestial art forms! The frequency and the vibration found within the perimeter of the circle are higher than that outside of the circle.

The vibration these Crop Circles carry is another form of light. Since it is unseen, it can be referred to, for all intents and purposes, as some form of "black light". These Crop Circles are thus, magnificent representations of these force fields of unseen or black light. But, it doesn't stop there. The vibration is not only higher within, but various experiments show that its vibrational frequency places a signature on the very seeds of the plants within the circle. These seeds mimic the same vibrational rate and continue to duplicate themselves and grow their offspring with this special vibrational signature. We are the seed producers of a New Paradigm of Healing Warriors. The more who gather within these circles, the higher our frequency will be. The more we change the way we think, the greater the seed production and thus, the greater chance for us to duplicate ourselves. Don't worry about being the "only one" in any City on this Planet, as your being there is as a seed planted in good soil. In fact, the "dirtier" the environment in your city, the greater your ability to grow and to crop and raise up New Seed Warriors of this Healing Mission! Don't be Afraid, Go Ahead and Duplicate Yourself! Let's not waste any more time. Go to Work!

Collectively, Beautiful Ones, we are calling the soldiers of the Most High to gather by the waters given to us through this New Paradigm of change. We are being called to gather and form these Crop Circles of "blacklight". We are being called to Duplicate the light that is within our circles and to spread this light to all! Awaken the sleeping lions and call them to life! Don't be afraid of yourself. Let's Do This! Today is our Day! We are Children of the Most High. We are Warriors of the Black Light... Rise up! Reclaim Your Name and Your Fame!

Ashe!
~*Dr Tisa Muhammad, Visionary Founder of: A Phoenix Rising Wellness Institute*

From Circles To Spirals

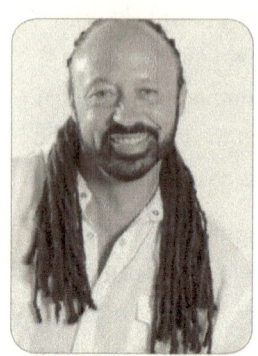

Katriel Wise is a metaphysical musical medicine man. His life song is to awaken humanity to its infinite potential using the tremendous, healing power of music. Katriel uses sound to manifest transformation of planet Earth. As a recording artist, songwriter and producer he has worked with Stevie Wonder and Patti Labelle to name a few. A vocalist and instrumentalist on flutes, saxophones, aboriginal Australian didgeridoo, Native and African drums, he blends his soulful roots with various genres such as jazz, reggae, soul, world and meditative. This musical alchemy creates a healing affect which repairs and regenerates the listener's spiritual DNA.

Katriel writes: **Elevating From Circles To Spirals.** *Western civilization has been in a linear, patriarchal and logic- oriented mode for several thousand years and thus has dominated the world through conquest. Now the return of the matriarch brings circular creativity and compassion. The next level is SPIRAL which is reflected throughout nature and music. It is not enough to be circular because a circle can be caught in a loop that can't elevate to its fullest potential. When musical notes are played the pattern is circular, yes, but the harmonics of the overtones ascend in spiral patterns. Likewise, when we make the conscious choice to eat foods in their original whole form, the spirals are visible to the eye. Try it yourself. Cut open an orange, okra, celery base …on & on to infinity….. notice the spiral patterns…. Heal thyself starting in a Circle of Wellness and daily, as you do the work of wellness, witness yourself holistically ascending into a spiral of profound transformation. THE NEW STAR GENERATION CAN ALSO BE CALLED THE SPIRAL GENERATION*

*In Love & Oneness…***Katriel**

Contact: stepwise9@gmail.com or (484) 410-WISE (9473)
Visit: http://www.stepwiseentertainment.com & www.wisdompreserve.land

DIVINE IS WITHIN YOU

by Stephen Wise

It's an illusion to believe that this is all we are
When it's a fact that we originated from the stars
And like the song that says "Your dreams will take you very far"
Soon you will know

That you can travel anywhere below or up above
Or stop a hurricane from destroying the ones you love
Bring to your life all of the joy that you've been dreaming of
When you go inside..........

Divine is within you Divine is within me too
Know anything you ask will be fulfilled if you're sincere
That pure intention is your power when you have no fear
So go within because the time to shine your light is here
All throughout the world

A sacred temple is our body when we realize
That eating living food is when we feel the most alive
And immortality is knowing you don't have to die,
We don't have to die..........

Divine is within you Divine is within me too

TRANSFORMATION

by Stephen "Katriel" Wise

Unison
    Transformation
    I'm ready for a change
    My destination

Harmony
    To a higher place

In The Spirit Of Transformation

In the spirit of transformation and preservation, Queen Afua suggests engaging in further research of Ken Keyes, Jr.:

> "When enough of us are aware of something, all of us become aware of it…we have the power to make changes if we can join together and raise our voices in unison. There is more power in numbers…let our numbers grow exponentially as we all take it on ourselves to spread these messages. We are the bearers of a new vision. We can dispel the old destructive myths and replace them with the life-enriching truths that are essential to continued life on our planet."

(As was transcribed from **The Hundredth Monkey,** by Ken Keyes, Jr., a book with the following copyright information: LIBRARY OF CONGRESS CATALOG NO. 81-70978 / ISBN 0-942024-01-X. This book is not copyrighted. You are asked to reproduce it in whole or in part, to distribute it with or without charge, in as many languages as possible, to as many people as possible. The rapid alerting of all humankind to nuclear realities is supremely urgent. If we are wiped out by nuclear destruction in the next few years, how important are the things we are doing today?)

Queen Afua

Welcome To The Catalogue
Of
Products & Services
Courses & Workshops
and
Entrpenuretial Opportunities
Offered At
The Queen Afua Wellness Center

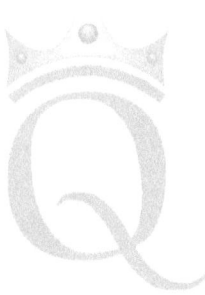

Please call or email:
Tel: 888.344.HEAL (4325)
feedback@queenafua.com
visit: www.queenafua.com

QUEEN AFUA WELLNESS STORE
QUEEN AFUA WELLNESS ONLINE STORE - WWW.QUEENAFUA.COM

Formulas

Green Life Formula 1
Master Herbal formula 2
Colon Inner Ease Formula 3
Herbal Laxative Formula 4
Supa Mega Green Formula

Rejuvenation clay Formula 5
Breath of life formula 6
Woman's Life Formula 7
Men's Life Formula 8

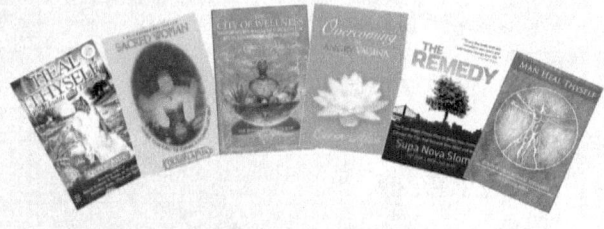

Books

Heal Thyself
Sacred Woman
City of Wellness
Overcoming an Angry Vagina
The Remedy
Man Heal Thyself

Wellness Charts

Nutrition Kitchen
Pyramid of Wellness
City OF Wellness Roadmap
Holistic/Vibrant Children

Womb Yoga
City of Wellness Chakra/Akrit
Womb Wisdom
Hydrotherapy Bath Spa Chart

Scrolls

Woman Heal Thyself
Man Heal Thyself
Hydrotherapy Bath Spa

Empowerment CD Consultations

21 Day Roadmap to Optimal Wellness
Mental and Nervous System Wellness
Respiratory Wellness
Bone and Joint Wellness
Colon Wellness
Blood and Circulatory Wellness

Womb Wellness
Prostate Wellness
Breast Wellness
Emotional Wellness
Pancreatic Wellness
Vibrant Youthful Skin

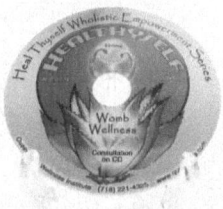

DVD's

Womb Yoga Dance
Holistic Wellness for the Hip Hop Generation

*Inquire for Sacred Woman Gateway Kits and Man Heal Thyself Kits
Tools for Body, Mind and Spirit Transformation

WELLNESS CHARTS

The Liberation Diet Pyramids of Wellness
Within five minutes of viewing the chart, one is instantly clear on how to heal thyself. you will be amazed at how quickly You and your family achieve holistic wellness.

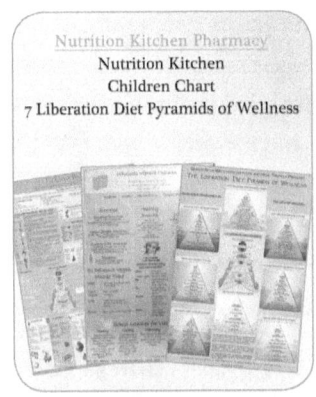

Nutrition Kitchen Pharmacy
Nutrition Kitchen
Children Chart
7 Liberation Diet Pyramids of Wellness

Nutrition Kitchen Chart
This chart is the wave of the future for healthy radiant citizens of wellness. This chart gives you food as medicine wellness

Tools to restore your body temple into wholeness. The chart includes the Liberation Menu Plan, natural food alternative shopping list, common kitchen herbs for healing, and the relationship of the seven kitchens of consciousness to the body's anatomy. From Flexitarian seeker of wellness to vegetarian/vegan devotee to raw food activist, this chart is sure to enlighten you.

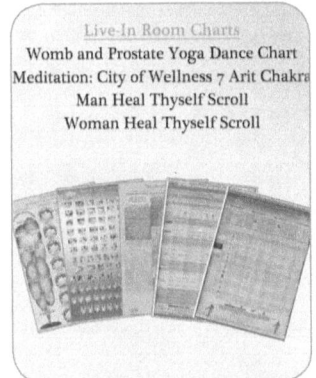

Live-In Room Charts
Womb and Prostate Yoga Dance Chart
Meditation: City of Wellness 7 Arit Chakra
Man Heal Thyself Scroll
Woman Heal Thyself Scroll

The Road Map to Optimal Wellness Chart
This chart will inspire one to not only get on the journey to wellness, but to maintain wellness as a way of life, to secure a healthy body, mind and spirit. Walk this Emerald Life. Invest time, energy, vision, and resources to build your inner city of vitality and witness every aspect as your being, Heal Thyself.

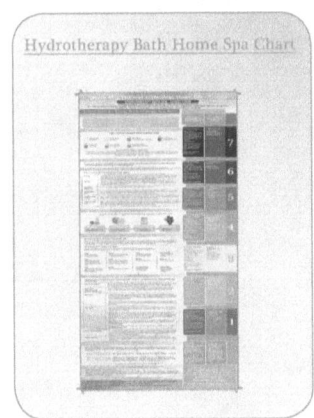

Hydrotherapy Bath Home Spa Chart

7 Arit City of Wellness Chart

The seven Arits are energy vortexes of vitality which through affirmation, visualization, contemplation, meditation and journaling, you will be able to purify and harmonize your psycho-physical-spiritual body. Take five to fifteen minutes to meditate, daily and elevate your inner Wellness.

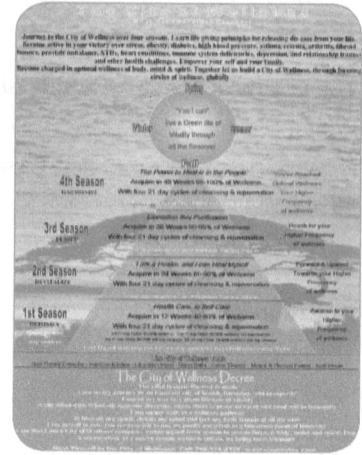

Holistic Vibrant Children Chart

This wellness chart supports children for living a holistic lifestyle. It offers child friendly, healthy morning fruit smoothies, vegan lunches and suppers,. It offers nature remedies for children in order to help parents raise vibrant youth.

Services, Consultations & Therapies

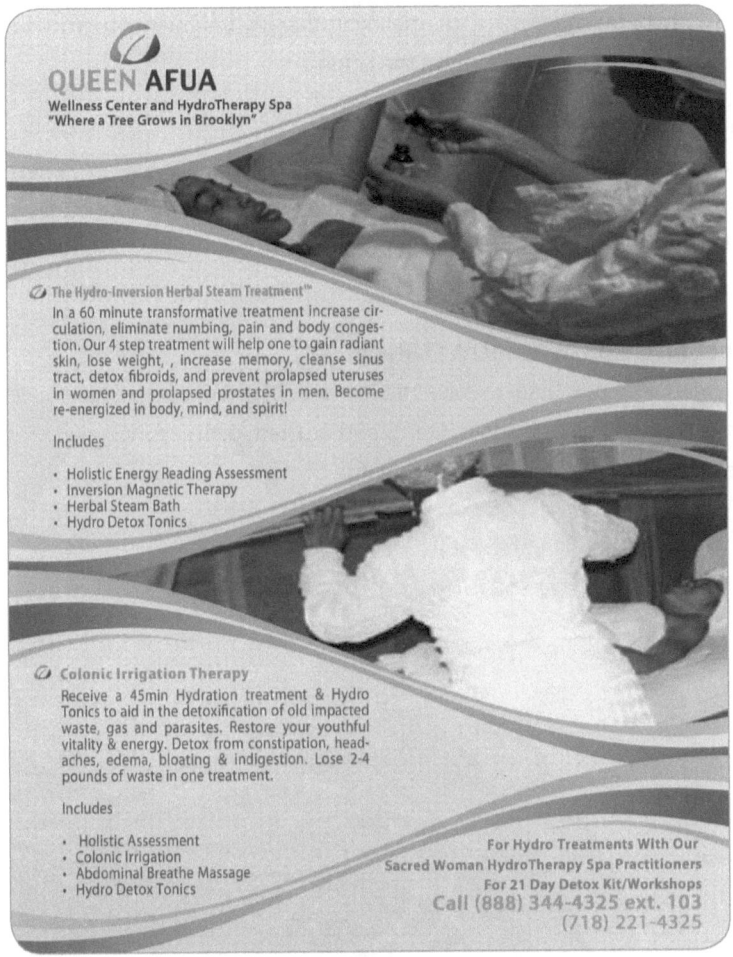

21 Day Holistic Lifestyle Consultations

Challenged with high blood pressure, stress, headaches, pain, depression, obesity, prostate issues, erectile dysfunction, fibroid tumors and other dis-eases? For radiant health, easy weight loss, full body rejuvenation and detoxification, sign up for a 1-hour private consultation for your particular needs.

Colon Wellness Hydrotherapy Treatment

Challenged with constipation, gas and abdominal bloating? Come in for a series of (30-45 minute) colonics; an internal hydrotherapy treatment to remove old impacted waste and parasites from the colon.

Herbal Detox Sweat

Challenged with stress, psoriasis, eczema, acne, boils or skin issues? Refresh your life and rest inside of a dome-shaped sweat chamber for 30 minutes as you detoxify and revitalize your pores from head to toe with a master herbal compound

Magnet Inversion Movement Therapy

Challenged with numbing, circulation blockage, blocked arteries, headaches, stress, prolapsed colon, bladder, uterus and prostate concerns? Come in for an Inversion Session and rejuvenate your entire anatomy.

Queen Afua Wellness Center

presents

The Circle of Wellness

Training Catalogue

Circles Of Wellness

Master Transformation Workshop

1 Day Detox Retreat
In your Home, City, Country
with Queen Afua as Your Guide

Circles of Wellness: A Guide to Planting, Cultivating & Harvesting Wellness is Queen Afua's newest book. Released in 2015, it includes 5 chapters of *Paradigm Shifts* which encourage participants to gather together at the Global Round Table in the home and community to make balanced, graceful transitions to the freedom of healthy living. It provides an opportunity to rethink and redo our personal and planetary health care. *"Health Care Is Self Care"*

Become fearless with your wellness. Make a paradigm shift into a Circle of Wellness; transform your entire life and the lives of all your relations. Queen Afua's newly released book, *Circles of Wellness: A Guide* is a guide to help end individual, community and planetary suffering and dis-ease and therefore bring about sustainable holistic living. This book is a master plan to holistically empower, "We, the People".

The teaching of the text is a call-out for "change", to take humanity off the collision course of dis-ease, disharmony and violence. *Circles of Wellness* will embark you on a freedom pathway to wellness for mental, physical, spiritual and relationship healing. The teachings in this book are to help you recognize that you have already created the power that circles you. The teachings are presented to get every individual, every family and every global community to a safe haven.

Each person can learn to live in circles to raise your frequency. You can learn how to set up Wellness Healing Homes, how to come into personal power center circles and learn to use the Empowerment Circle Wheels to assist your family and community to overcome health challenges.

Become a Holistic Caretaker. Save your greatest treasures: yourself, your children and your elders in a Circle of Wellness. Heal Thyself and become a holistic community activist for change. Together we can end mental, emotional, physical and social disease. Holistically, we can break the addictive chains of unhealthy living. We each can wake up our inner healer and all together can make a paradigm shift to a global world of peace and vitality.

Sponsor Queen Afua
Seminars, Workshops, Keynotes, Retreats
Become a Circle of Wellness Host
for your family, spiritual house, community, city, country

For reservations:
888-344-HEAL (4325) x 107
Email: bookings@queenafua.com

Emerald Green 21 Day Detox Courses:

Level 1. Personal Detox

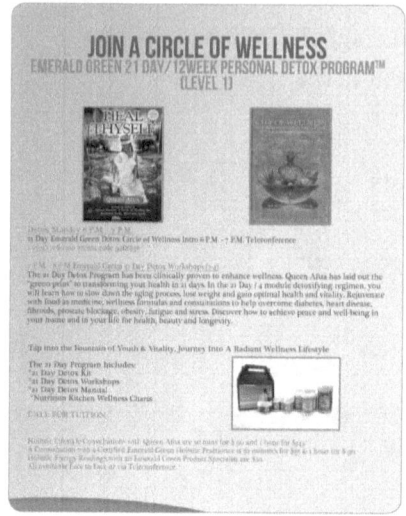

Level 2. Product Consultant

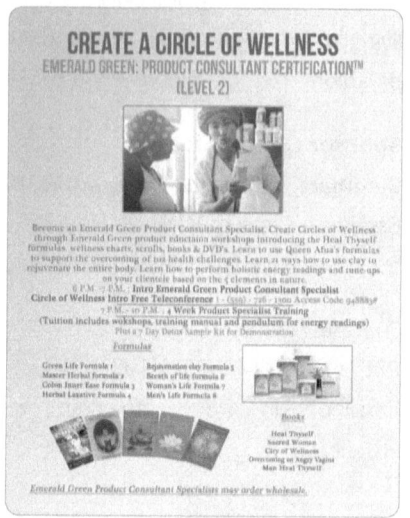

Level 3. Advanced Practitioner Certification

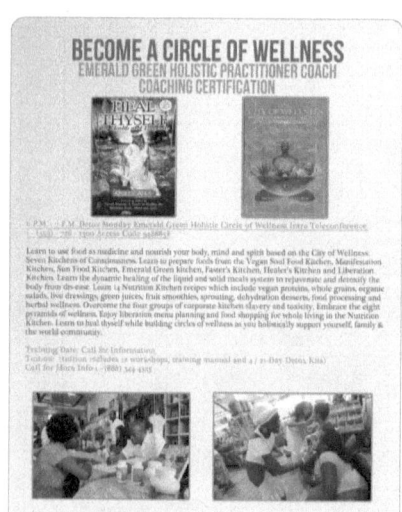

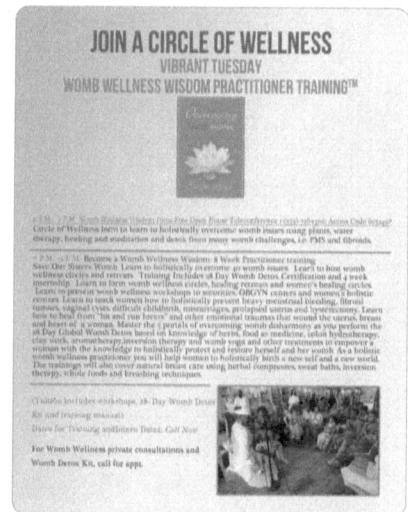

Queen Afua's signature 21-Day Detox programs are based on texts she authored. Her first book **Heal Thyself: For Health & Longevity** provides both men and women the opportunity to awaken the healer within in 21 days. Further training is based on **The City of Wellness: Restoring Your Health Through the Seven Kitchens of Consciousness** which initiated the City

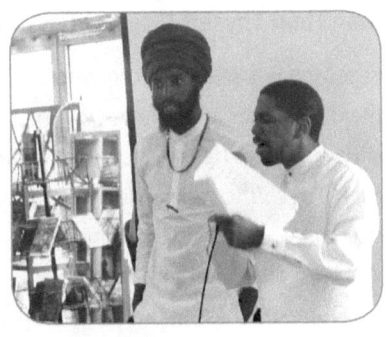

of Wellness campaign which reminds us that we do not have to live with pain, dis-ease and fear. Individuals can learn to observe the relationship between their food lifestyle and their wellness. Participants enjoy liberation menu planning and food shopping guidelines for whole living in the Nutrition Kitchen Pharmacy.

Rites of Passage Training Courses:

Sacred Woman Rites of Passage Training Course

Queen Afua coaches Women into balance and alignment within their spiritual anatomy through the Gateways of her best-selling Sacred Woman Text Book. Contents include: Sacred Movement, beauty, relationship and intuitive healing by the usage of plants, flower essences, color therapy, gemstone healing, element healing, meditation, affirmations and music to restore and harmonize the feminine body, mind and spirit. This course is for guiding women towards healthier relationships with each other and all of their relations.

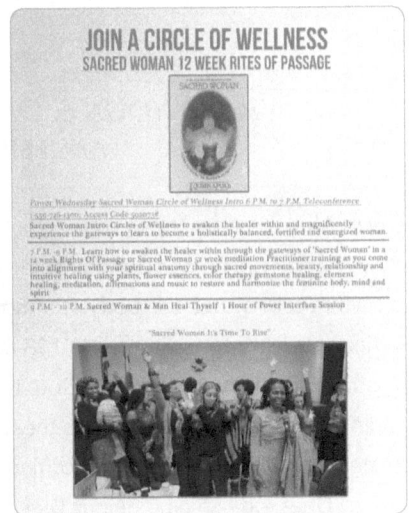

Man Heal Thyself Rites of Passage Training Course

Based on her years of experiencing the imbalances in women, Queen Afua produces her newest work, **Man Heal Thyself** to guide Men towards becoming Heal Thyself Wellness Warriors. Designed to help men to maximize wellness and restore the heart, lower blood pressure, prevent diabetes, heal prostate illness and release "The Five Wounded Men" within and discover the inner Wellness Warrior. Men and Women come together in harmony to heal each other and the entire family, producing a wellness community, city and eventually a healthier world.

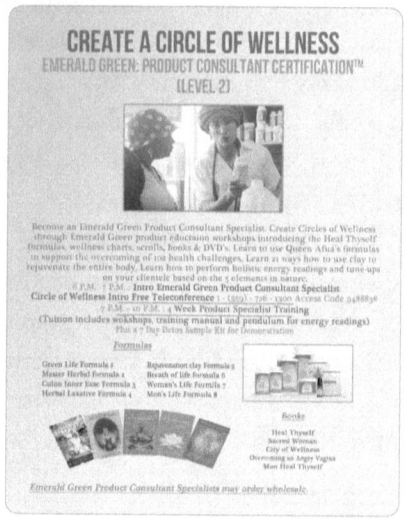

WOMB YOGA & DANCE OF THE WOMB MASTER CLASSES

Queen Afua presents The Womb Yoga Dance! Lean 69 Womb Yoga poses to harmonize the body, mind and spirit and 39 Womb Yoga Dance poses to rhythmically attune the body as a moving temple of peace and serenity. Participants learn to master these 108 movements to strengthen align and empower the body, bringing the Soul to Life. Study the mystical transformative healing language of Queen Afua's theatrical production, *Dance of the Womb*, created, choreographed and performed by Queen Afua, inspired by ancient African Ones –the Shining Beings Dwelling in Light.

For tuition and schedule call: 888-344-HEAL (4325)

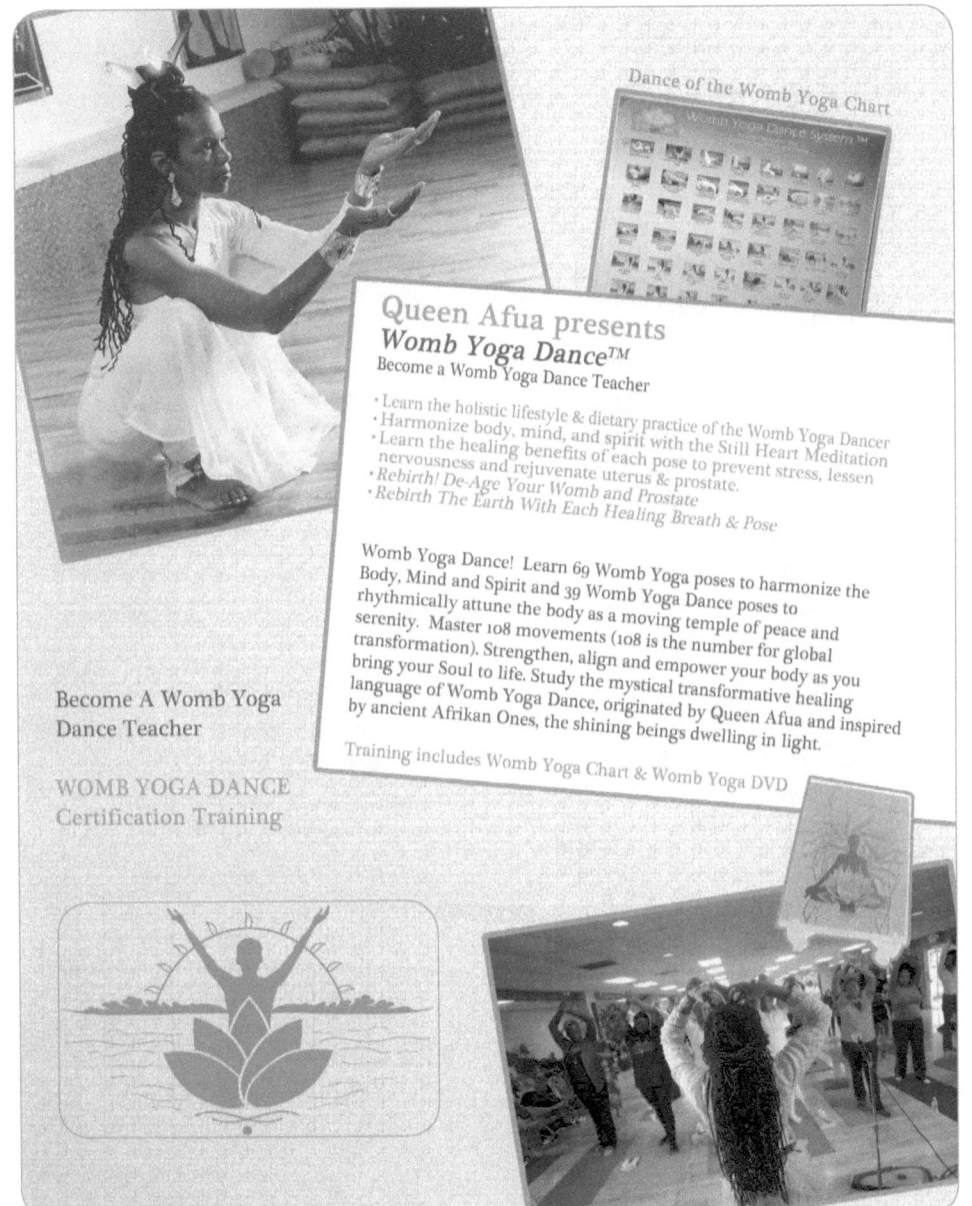

ONGOING...

*W*e are gathered at this Global Round Table because everything we need is here, in this circle there is something for everyone...

When we are in harmony with nature, we are in harmony with ourselves. Healthy people can look forward to creating healthy relationships. In Circles of Wellness, we can begin to end violence in the home and violence in the world. People in Circles of Wellness, can formulate creative solutions for transforming our global wellness one person, one circle and one community at a time.

Fellow Humans, we are gathered here at the Global Round Table facing worldwide challenges and facing each other. It is our time to be victorious in our journey toward Global Wellness and Global Harmony.

In closing **Circles of Wellness,** I sat with my most devoted, youthful (*but ancient*) student, Quasheba Shamla El-Dey. While I wrote and she typed, we reflected back and forth the final words in Circles. Sunset grew near; Quasheba, (the voice of the future) had an "Ah, ha" moment, *"Don't Push The Button. Every day our cellular nuclei are being attacked on the mental, physical and spiritual levels. This is the true Nuclear war. Every time you push the button on a vending machine, pull up at the drive-thru window, hang up the phone on someone in need or eat GMO foods, a multidimensional missile is launched. Nuclear war is a metaphor for what is happening to us on the cellular levels. The nucleus of a cell is the center of all its activity. This is reflected in the way that a woman is the nucleus of a family and the family is the nucleus of a community. As we build up our circles we will build a strong force field that will protect us from Nuclei Destruction."*

Think about it. This is the paradigm shift.

With all my heart,

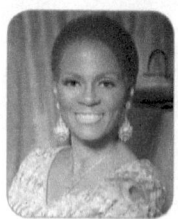

Queen Afua

THE POWER TO HEAL IS WITHIN US!

www.ingramcontent.com/pod-product-compliance
Lightning Source LLC
Chambersburg PA
CBHW020737180526
45163CB00001B/270